- Dec 2001
  $15⁰⁰
- Outdoor
  Life
- Reference
  manual

The National Outdoor Leadership School's

# Wilderness Guide

## THE CLASSIC HANDBOOK, REVISED AND UPDATED

## MARK HARVEY

A FIRESIDE BOOK
PUBLISHED BY SIMON & SCHUSTER

FIRESIDE
Rockefeller Center
1230 Avenue of the Americas
New York, NY 10020

FIRESIDE and colophon are registered trademarks
of Simon & Schuster Inc.

Designed by Chris Welch
Illustrations by Rick Ruhman

Manufactured in the United States of America
10  9  8  7  6  5  4  3  2  1

Library of Congress Cataloging-in-Publication Data
Harvey, Mark W. T. (Mark William Thornton)
    The National Outdoor Leadership School's wilderness guide : the
classic handbook / Mark Harvey. —Rev. and updated.
        p.  cm.
    Rev. ed. of: The National Outdoor Leadership School's wilderness
guide / Peter Simer. ©1983
    "A Fireside book."
    Includes bibliographical references and index.
    1. Backpacking.  2. Camping.  3. Wilderness survival.  4. National
Outdoor Leadership School (U.S.)  I. Simer, Peter, 1947—  National
Outdoor Leadership School's wilderness guide.  II. Title.
III. Title: Wilderness guide.
GV199.6.S56      1999
796.51'028—dc21                                    99-21875
                                                      CIP

ISBN 0-684-85909-2

This book is dedicated with admiration and affection to the men and women at NOLS who give so generously of themselves in teaching students to love and care for the wilds.

And it is dedicated with gratitude to the two people who gave me countless opportunities and kept me on the straight and narrow, Connie Harvey and the memory of Harold K. Harvey.

# Contents

## Chapter 6: Travel Technique     134

## Chapter 7: Leadership and Expedition Behavior     165

## Chapter 8: Maps and Compasses     178

# Chapter 9: Emergency Procedures    203

# Chapter 10: Weather    215

# List of Figures

# Acknowledgments

This book attempts to capture the outdoor philosophy and techniques of the National Outdoor Leadership School and therefore credit should go to the many staff members and instructors (beginning with founder Paul Petzoldt) who have made the school what it is today.

Many people helped to produce this book. My thanks for the invaluable assistance, ideas, and encouragement from the NOLS review committee: Jim Ferguson, John Gookin, Lannie Hamilton, Phil Powers, Tom Reed, and Liz Alva Rosa.

Molly Doran, Tod Shimelpfenig, Kevin McGowan, Drew Leemon, and Rich Brame offered excellent suggestions in their areas of expertise.

Four readers outside NOLS helped me very much with the manuscript: Joan McCarter, Ann Harvey, Connie Harvey, and John Katzenberger.

Thanks to my agent, Michael Congdon, for his help in all aspects of the production of this book. Thanks to Molly Hampton, NOLS director of personnel, for her help in launching this project in the early stages.

I am grateful to the executive director of NOLS, John Gans, and the NOLS board of trustees for their support of the project.

At Simon & Schuster, I would like to thank Sarah Baker, Betsy Radin-Herman, Bette Alexander, and Matt Walker for their skillful editing and management of the production process.

Thank you John Roskelley, Pamela Eaton, Jeff Foott, Molly Doran, Buck Tilton, and Sam Talucci for taking the time to be interviewed.

To Rick Ruhman, my appreciation for your hard work on the illustrations.

Finally, I am very grateful to Molly Absolon for her tremendous skills and constant support in all stages of the production of this book—thanks, Molly!

# Foreword

Have you ever wondered what it would be like to live self-sufficiently on the snow and ice of Alaska's big peaks? Or paddle a sea kayak into the limitless expanse of the Patagonian coast? Maybe you're dying to learn how to climb sheer granite walls in the wilds of Wyoming or probe hidden grottoes in Utah's slickrock country. NOLS can help you thrive in these places. NOLS will teach you how to flourish in the wilderness without impacting it, how to lead your peers with competence. From moving with the tides of Baja in a kayak to living comfortably above timberline in the Rockies, NOLS enables such dreams to become self-sustaining realities.

One can't tell the story of the National Outdoor Leadership School without mentioning its founder, Paul Petzoldt. In 1965, Petzoldt, who had made a name for himself climbing mountains, training World War II troops, and teaching outdoor skills, tackled his most ambitious project in a lifetime full of lofty accomplishments. In that year, Petzoldt founded the National Outdoor Leadership School in Lander, a small west-central Wyoming town that few people outside the state had ever heard of. But Lander was (and is) the perfect location for a school designed to teach leadership and wilderness skills. Outside the front door of Petzoldt's school lay the fabulous Wind River Range, a spine of granite and ice and wilderness stretching more than 100 miles across the state. The Winds were a perfect classroom for Petzoldt, and his ambitious project soon became a reality. Students came to Lander to learn such things as how to camp without leaving a trace, how to rock climb, how to stay warm and dry in the wilderness, what to do in case of an emergency, and how to lead. They learned a lot more too, much of which wasn't even in the curriculum. They learned how to communicate with one another, how to "roll with the punches" on a hard day, and how to back off when they were in over their heads.

Today, the National Outdoor Leadership School is the leader in wilderness education. Since Petzoldt's modest start in 1965, the school has expanded and grown, reaching out to more than 50,000 people worldwide. New classrooms have been added around the globe, from Patagonia to Arizona, Alaska to Mexico, East Africa to Australia. People have turned to NOLS to learn many things, and they've discovered a lot about themselves in the process. A NOLS course teaches students how to live and travel in the backcountry with minimal impact on the environment. A typical course is a month long and filled with adventures, challenges, and interesting people. Leadership is an integral part of all courses. Skills taught in NOLS courses run the gamut from mountaineering, rock climbing, sea kayaking, horsepacking, backpacking, caving, telemark skiing, canoeing, sailing, whitewater rafting, kayaking, and canyoneering. Such skills are the hands-on, practical stuff that a student learns by doing, not by plotting out some theory in triangles and squares in a textbook. That's what NOLS is all about, and in many ways, that's what this book is all about.

NOLS is still located in Lander, Wyoming, at the foot of the Winds, but the school has evolved a great deal from the early days. First and foremost, NOLS is a school—with a curriculum and educators—that offers college credit. The school has formed vital public and private partnerships such as the international Leave No Trace program, an effort to bring the minimum impact camping ethic to popular attention. NOLS has a research arm, a fundraising branch, an endowment, scholarships, a marketing department, class textbooks and publications. *The NOLS Wilderness Guide* was first published in 1983 by Peter Simer and John Sullivan. Simer, the former executive director for NOLS, and Sullivan graciously passed the baton to NOLS instructor and author Mark Harvey for this refurbished edition.

We hope you'll find this revised and updated version of *The Wilderness Guide* indispensable to your wilderness adventures. Mark Harvey has accumulated and compiled knowledge from more than three decades and made it understandable, even poetic at times. You should use this book as a tool, not as a crutch. In these pages, you'll learn about weather and cooking, backpacking gear and wilderness travel. But, again, don't be just an armchair traveler. As we do in all NOLS courses, we encourage you to get out there and, as Nike says, "Just do it." Our alumni have done just that. They've come to the school, learned as much as they could possibly cram in, and have gone out and applied their new talents. Some of our graduates have used the wilderness skills time and again in a life spent outdoors. Others applied the leadership lessons to business and have been fabulously successful. Still more pause every once in a while, remembering that tawny, gentle quality of the last bit of sunlight on a high mountain peak, or the surreal liquid image of a whale just feet off their kayak bow, or simply a special friend with an addictive laugh. That's what NOLS is all about: the experience. We hope you'll use this book, learn the lessons, and then experience the experience. Enjoy our world's great wilderness, take care of it, and take care of yourself.

—Tom Reed, NOLS Publications Manager

For more information, contact The National Outdoor Leadership School at 288 Main Street, Lander, WY 82520, visit us on the Web at www.nols.edu, or call 307-332-5300.

# CHAPTER 1

# Why We Go

Nature is, after all, the great reservoir of energy, of confidence, of endless hope, and of that joy not wholly subdued by the pale cast of
thought. . . .

—*The Best Nature Writing of Joseph Wood Krutch*

Spring refuses to come to my corner of Colorado this year. It's mid-April
and this morning I awoke to a wet snow blizzard and suffocating gray
skies. The weather map shows no relief in sight. It's time to go to the
desert, a part of the world that seems to have a better understanding of the
seasons. I call a friend, a guy I can rely on for good conversation, and he
agrees that a trip to the desert is the only solution.

A couple of hours later we're on the highway driving west, Merle Haggard
on the radio singing about how to pull out of a tailspin when your world
buckles under the weight of a broken heart. I glance at my friend out of the
corner of my eye and he looks dodgy in the early morning light. He's un-
shaven, his eyes are bloodshot, and he's listening intently to Merle as if he's
going to pick up a gem of information. I worry about people when they listen too closely to Merle Haggard and I know my friend is lovesick these days.

The snow won't relent even after an hour of driving. My friend sits in a
dark, moody silence, and I'm beginning to have some doubts about this trip.
It's impossible not to start thinking about the comforts I've left behind in my
cozy cabin. Though I fancy myself an outdoorsman, I am also a product of
the twentieth century, and thus I have surrounded myself with all the amenities that make life comfortable. My cabin has central heating, I have a four-
wheel-drive truck that starts cheerfully on arctic mornings, my mattress

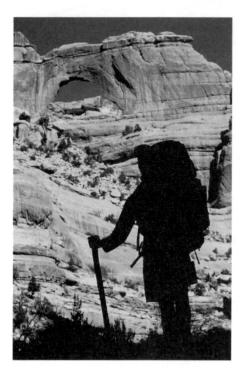

A NOLS student silhouetted in front of Neville's Arch in Owl Canyon, Utah, on a fall semester course. *John McConnell*

could keep any princess cushioned from the pea, I have a fast computer, and my stereo has acoustic fidelity. Life in my quarter of the civilized world is good and cushy. But every couple of weeks, I go into my camping closet— whose space occupies roughly a third of my cabin—put some gear together, find a friend with some free time, and strike out for the backcountry, where there are considerably fewer amenities and creature comforts.

Today, with the weather and its prospects, with the glum silence of my friend, I'm wondering why I ever left my house. At home I can control the ambient temperature of my cabin to within a degree or two. On this trip to the desert, I can't do anything about the ambient temperature and may have to suffer a bit if this snow continues. At home I can go to the supermarket and buy fresh fruit flown in from South America; if we want something fresh in the backcountry this week, we'll have to hunt or scavenge. At home I have headroom in my house and rows of books in my shelves. So why have I chosen to go live in a small tent with one book and an unsavory campmate who looks none too stable today? At first glance, the tradeoffs don't look good and in this light one might think it daft to surrender one square inch of the easeful life in the city for all things wild.

Maybe it is daft. What species besides humans chooses to leave a sheltered life for the rugged and harsh outback? Wild animals—elk, coyotes, bears, and the rest—go places where they can find the most forage and shelter, the most fish perhaps, or protected areas to calve their young. Wild animals do all they can to make their lives safer, fatter, and warmer, because otherwise they'll go hungry and even die. Reptiles, with their primitive thermostats, commute back and forth between the sun and the shade depending on the air temperature. But on weekends and vacations, you and I and millions of other people leave our safe, fat, and warm lives for the lean wilds. And we do so happily, without hopes of improving our footing in the material world. Surely there must be impressive reasons why we go.

You can sit in a library or lecture hall and learn wonderful things about how the Visigoths sacked Rome or about string theory and particle physics. But no library or university will show you how plants time their blooming over the course of a season, how a moose behaves or a skunk misbehaves, or how reptiles make a living from the poor pickings of the desert. Books and professors can describe these things but to really know them you have to see them with your own eyes. We go to the wilderness to learn things we can't learn from any academic treatise or self-help book. The wilds teach us things we can learn only there.

The wildlands teach us to be smart, practical, resourceful, and observant.

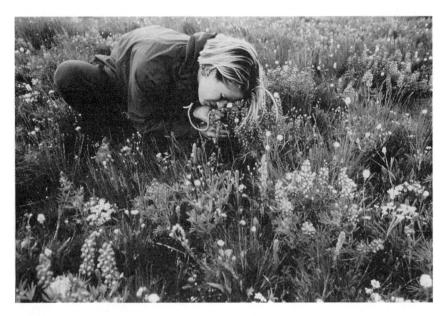

A NOLS student studies lupine flowers with a hand lens. *Whit Bronaugh*

To hike ten hours through scabrous terrain, cross a brawny river, stay warm in a snowstorm, and navigate your way out of tangled woods tests and builds your best faculties. The cities, in opposition, often teach us to be cunning, artful, and sly. In Washington, D.C., you can find your way out of a crisis with a spin doctor and a few evasions. You can answer questions with vagaries and nonanswers and still stay atop the heap. But the most artful sleight of hand won't get you down a steep ridge in a lightning storm; power games and paper trading won't help you cross the river and stay warm at night. Only your most honest and best traits will help you when you go out and test yourself in the wilds: judgment, patience, strength, and—dare I say this—character.

The jingoism of politics may have tinged and devalued the word *character*, but it's still a quality people understand and try to instill in their children. Character seems to come from hardship and difficulties and challenges. Sports, they say, build character. Heartbreak, they say, builds character. But nature insists on character. Roald Amundsen got to the South Pole because of his character—a weaker character wouldn't have made it past 70 degrees south. Lewis and Clark completed 2,000 miles and two years of rough travel to the Pacific not by wits alone, but with faith in themselves, the courage to embark on the unknown, and the flint to pick themselves up after failure—in short, through their depth of character. With today's schedules, it's hard to find two years to map a new continent, but we can bring our characters to bear even on a weekend's backpacking trip.

After four hours of driving, my friend and I finally arrive at the trailhead. We make the last-minute preparations with our gear, check a map, and finally light out to see the desert's mysteries. The first mile feels sluggish, the packs weigh heavy on our shoulders, and my friend continues his morbid silence. So far, I feel few of what John Muir called "nature's good tidings," and, maybe it's my imagination, but one of my boots seems to be rubbing a bit on the heel.

By the second mile, we have settled into a better rhythm and some of the desert's beauty is forcing itself onto us. It has rained here recently and the air is thick with the smells of bitterbrush, sage, and Mormon tea. The highway noise is receding and we are walking across that margin that separates the world dominated by man and industry from the world as it existed a million years ago. The adobe red sandstone dominates the landscape, and is broken only by clumps of juniper, piñon, and sage.

When we stop to rest after about an hour, my friend has some color back in his face and I can see the light is returning to his eyes. Still, he's barely said a word and the wistful look hasn't entirely left his face. We take a big chug of water from our water bottles and put our packs back on to continue into the desert.

We go to the backcountry to find the peace we can't find in the front country. In the front country, we've overbuilt our infrastructure and overheated our schedules, and we glory in the resulting frenzy. We toy with caffeine in the morning, commute distances that can't be sane, rush projects that were due yesterday, work late, and then wonder why our nights go sleepless.

In the wilds, you reduce your world to simple tasks like fetching water, pitching a tent, and cooking dinner. Sometimes it's as simple as putting one foot in front of the other. You are rewarded immediately for completing those tasks, not with a giddy buzz or a narcotic haze, but with the gratification of a pleasing meal, the warm shelter of a well-pitched tent, or a sublime view after scaling the heights of an alpine pass.

Once away from the whine of commerce and industry, you have the chance to let the business of your mind settle and puzzle out what this life means to you. Climb 3,000 feet up a canyon, even under the strain of a heavy backpack, and the petty company politics, the importance of being earnest, the inane things fall away like so much dead skin. Ah, clarity.

I suppose we go to the wilds to escape. We escape the urgent hullabaloo of the crowded world and that in itself is probably reason enough to go. The

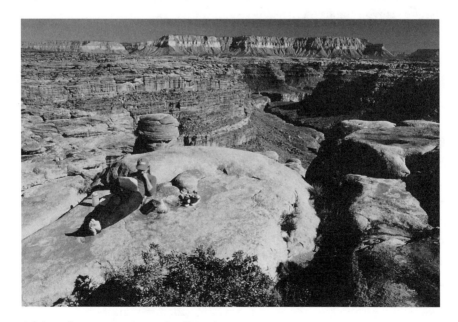

A hiker takes a rest in Canyonlands, Utah. *Glenn Goodrich*

wilds are a space where you come face to face with yourself and the stoic, impassive rhythms of the natural world. Some actually find the first couple of days in the mountains maddening without the stimulation of the cities. Separated from the action and ferment of the city, their hurried minds circle back upon themselves like tortured rats. Some bury their heads in a book or keep the Walkman deep in their ears to shut out the silence and repose. Sure, the wilds are an escape from the frenzy below, but the haste and charge of our modern lives are themselves an escape from the slower, deeper, resonating rhythms of nature. Our institutions and empires and laws, our marble columns, steel, and glass—what do they mean next to even a lowly pond with its primordial algae, stolid frogs, and the ticking insects?

Maybe we seek some sort of stability in a landscape that won't change faces. In an unsettling America we have all had favorite places that have been bought, divided, excavated, and developed into industrial parks or cookie-cutter housing strips. That can't happen in the wilds, we tell ourselves. When we look out over the canyons of the Southwest, paddle through the Boundary Waters of Minnesota, or hike in the Sierras, the land seems a solid point of reference that won't change in our lifetimes. If we have children, we show them places we knew as children and the landscape joins our lives. Governments can fall, the stock market can lose half its value, we can marry or divorce, find worldly success, fail miserably, or grow old, but something like the Grand Canyon stands there facing us forever.

Peaceful at times, nature is also raw and dangerous and thrilling. I have felt danger and excitement when two young bull moose lumbered across a meadow straight at me, wagging their impossibly large heads and antlers, menace in their step. I have felt afraid for my life crossing slopes with poor footing, gaping exposure, and thousands of feet of clear nothingness inviting just one slip, just one clumsy step. I have felt a mystifying calm when a lightning storm visited my camp high in the Rockies, and crashed and railed about us for what seemed hours. The woods are filled with worthy animals who nevertheless will bite and kick and sting if threatened. The weather, thank God, won't be controlled by science, and not all days sparkle and not all winds are gentle breezes. When you leave for the mountains, you try to travel safely and sensibly, but there is risk involved. In the wilds, you get to make battlefield decisions—shall we cross the pass in the lightning storm and maybe go up in a flash of fire or shall we hunker down and sit out the storm? That's what makes it vivid and exciting. The decisions out there call for boldness and clarity and usually go tested within a matter of hours.

We've probably hiked about five miles now, my friend and I, and I can feel the knots in my back and the cricks in my mind start to dissolve. I won't say the hiking is effortless—it's actually quite a grunt—but that nice hiker's trance that only comes of several hard miles has washed over me like a tonic. I feel I could hike forever.

A jackrabbit bolts from the sage and a red-tailed hawk tips its wings to have a look. But the rabbit is fleet and will live another day. The scenery and the desert fragrance must be getting the better of my friend because he finally breaks his silence with a comment on the plight of the jackrabbit and the predatory hawk, with an allusion to the writings of Leon Trotsky and the petit bourgeois. I am embarrassed that I don't understand the allusion, but happy that my friend is coming around. I know it will only take a few more miles of desert tramping before he's fully himself.

We go because the wilds are brutal and primeval and primordial and so, deep down, are we—at least a part of us. Call it the Id, if you like; call it the influence of the Dark Gods. In the wilds we can loosen up and unbend, shake the "galling harness of civilization," as John Muir put it, and no one will think us odd or commit us to the padded institutions: fortunately, those who would commit us don't bother to leave the cities. Out in the wilderness we have to fight harder for our survival and engage the robust qualities that got us through millions of years of evolution. The woods are a welcome relief to that stifled part of our animal being. We are, in a sense, walking the dog—that wild dog in us who doesn't like the civilization below. What grim creator would have us develop as rough animals for an eternity and then forever restrict us to the norms of polite society?

Oddly enough, the wilderness is one of the best places to make friends and even fall in love. Perhaps it's because we depend on each other when we go to the woods or the mountains. We depend on each other in the cities, but it's not always quite so clear who relies on whom. Coming down a too-tricky ridge in the mountains, watch yourself develop a sudden affection for your more competent, catlike partner. Or if you're the agile one, you'll find yourself coaxing and nursing your clumsy friend to better footing. The elements and the many demands of raw nature force us to work together, to depend on each other. There are a thousand situations out there that call for us to depend on our teammates or, by turns, to extend a hand. If I'm exhausted, cold, and hungry, I'll need you to bring up my morale and you damn well better make a good dinner. If you've got a headache from the altitude, leave the thinking to me.

Our intrigue with nature is innate. Nature is not something that we need to be coached to love. To support this idea, I offer the development of children. My two-year-old nephew, for instance, has a fascination with horses against which not even the most garish toys or gooiest ice cream can com-

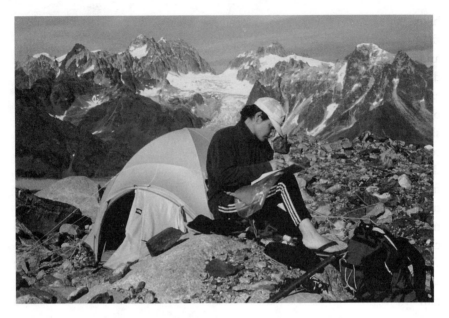

NOLS instructor Deborah Sussex taking a moment to write in her journal while teaching a mountaineering course in the Central Alaska Range. *Theo Singelis*

pete. The horse's otherness, its crudely shaped head, velvet lips, musky smells, and low murmur mesmerize him. The horse is the boy's center of reference, and when he can't work out the world, he points at the corral and mutters "Horsey, horsey, horsey." The boy is young enough that his mind is clear and hungry, his reactions to the world innate, not affected. In the cyber world, you might say his brain is unformatted. Why, then, has the horse, and increasingly now the cow, so "other than" human, become his center? His engrossment with a species not his own is, ironically, what makes him human and nudges us toward the reasons why nature is so important to our minds, souls, sanity, and life itself.

It should come as no surprise that the wilds bewitch his young mind and the human spirit. Despite our Italian colognes and top-heavy résumés, we are not so many years out of the woods. Surely an ancient portion of our consciousness has survived the 10,000 years of civilization and craves to wander through the forest once again. When you stack up the millions of years of our development in which we were just clever animals in nature against the few hundred years since we have effectively isolated ourselves from it, it's reasonable that we need to go back to the wilds to resuscitate our lives.

A short four days later my friend and I are driving back home at dusk. We hiked hard today to get back to the truck so we could return to our duties in the parallel world. I feel a nice weariness in my bones from the hard hiking and a quiet mind from whatever it is that the desert does after even a few days' visit. The changes are subtle, but seeing the scrappy creatures—the ravens, hawks, lizards, and snakes—going about their lives in this hardscrabble country is somehow comforting. The enormous landscape and infinite sky, so indifferent to our passage and so indifferent to the passage of time, are reassuring as well. It's George Jones who is singing on the radio now, about the misery of knowing his woman is in the arms of another. I check on my friend out of the corner of my eye for his reaction, worried that the wistful tune and melancholy lyrics will throw him back into his heavy-hearted trance. But he's too busy rambling on about our next trip to even hear the cheatin' song—ahh, the restorative effects of the desert.

Joseph Wood Krutch tells us that the fourteenth-century Italian poet and scholar Francesco Petrarch was the first who admitted to climbing a mountain just for the benefit of its view. Upon descending, according to some, he promptly apologized for his droll climb. But why apologize? Surely you have your own reasons for going to the wilds. The purpose of this book is really not to answer the "why," but rather to help with the "how." In this book we try to teach techniques that will make your trips more enjoyable, safer, more efficient, and, yes, more stylish. There is intrinsic value to camping well, but more important, camping well allows you to enjoy the wilds the way you want. And camping well helps you preserve the wilds for your next trip, for a trip your grandson or niece may make someday, and for the trip some total stranger will make without you ever knowing it. Camping well helps preserve the land for the very creatures that live there: the wild things. The techniques and ideas in this book certainly aren't the only ways to travel in the mountains. But they are good techniques used by many good outdoorspeople. Use this book to expand your own skills. Choose the techniques that work best for you. Above all, find the time to get out there.

# A Word About NOLS

I took my first NOLS course while still a freshman at college. I came to the course with none of the fire and gumption that I like to see in my own students nowadays as an instructor; rather, I was a trifle lost and unhappy with the world. When I finished the course, I had no intention of becoming an instructor and I'm sure the school had no intention of inviting me to apply for a position. But I did come away from the course on my feet, stronger for the experience, and with renewed interest in the world. I also came away impressed by the logic of the instruction and principles taught while we sea kayaked for three weeks. The skills that my instructors taught me were practical—even elegant—and carefully shorn of froufrou.

The skills are not unique to NOLS: There are lots of people in the world who know how to camp and travel expertly. But I think NOLS has been particularly good in developing a broad body of efficient principles that can be applied to the situation at hand, and then teaching them to others. In my opinion, the most important lesson taught on NOLS courses is *to use your brain*. NOLS instructors put it a little more delicately and say, "Use your judgment." Should you ever take a NOLS course you will likely hear that phrase a dozen times. Ask your NOLS instructor where to pitch a tent on the fourth night out on a course, and it's unlikely that he or she will suggest a site. Rather, you will be encouraged to choose your own campsite based on what you've learned about safety, minimum-impact camping, and perhaps the habits of bears—if you're in that sort of territory. In short, you'll be encouraged to develop and exercise good judgment every day of the course, so you have the tools to make decisions for yourself.

Good judgment comes from lots of experience but also from reflection on that experience. The nonthinking person will repeat the same mistake over and over and all the experience in the world won't teach him good judgment. The person who stops to reflect on what he has learned from each success and each failure can rapidly develop good judgment.

Later in this book we will talk about packs and tents and boots—all important items—but the single most important piece of equipment you have sits squarely above your shoulders, has two lobes, and a component that rhymes with *Gore-Tex:* call it your brain. In some ways our brains are highly overdeveloped, but in other ways they go untapped. I have been amazed to see people with little experience plan and execute a difficult evacuation, purposefully navigate their way out of nebulous terrain, or skillfully resolve personal conflicts. What is impressive about their successes is that despite their lack of experience, they take the time to think things through before acting—they use their brains. The unfortunate corollary is that many people abandon their senses in these same crises and end up turning a merely poor circumstance into a disaster.

Sometimes in the outdoors you just have to puzzle things out for yourself. You could memorize this book and a dozen more like it, but you will still have to use your judgment and your brain. We can teach the principles of how and when to cross a river, but when push comes to shove, you will have to make the tough decisions out there for yourself.

Consequently, it's important to give your brain a fighting chance by feeding it the best information available through experience, conversations with others, and reading books like this one.

Nature selects for good judgment because those with spectacularly poor judgment—those who light a smoke at the gas pump, perhaps—are mercifully plucked from the gene pool. The fact that you have to use your brain and use it well in the outdoors is at once part of the appeal and part of the discomfort.

Teaching good judgment and good tools to support that judgment has been the school's business for thirty years. It is the purpose of this book to share with you some of the same principles and techniques that NOLS has used to instruct tens of thousands of competent wilderness travelers over the last three decades.

# CHAPTER 2

# Expedition Planning

When the directors of the NOLS Patagonia branch plan a seventy-day semester, their decisions involve kayaks, horses, planes, boats, trucks, thousands of pounds of food, high expectations, unknown terrain, glaciers, devilish Patagonia weather, and even a tactfully written letter to the Chilean navy. The logistics for these trips are formidable, but the principles for planning them are the same principles you or I can use to plan a three-day trip to the Smoky Mountains.

The celebrated adventurer Bill Tilman once said, "Any worthwhile expedition can be planned on the back of an envelope." Expedition planning needn't be overly complex or metaphysical. Part of the fun of the outdoors comes in spontaneous trips when you call a few friends, throw some things in a pack, and head for the hills. But paradoxically, the people most successful at "spontaneous" trips are those with the practical experience to bring the right gear, some maps, and enough fuel, and the leadership experience to choose the right people for the venture—even if they leave for the wilds on the spur of the moment.

In the summer of 1998, Neal Beidleman, a guide credited with saving many lives on the ill-fated 1996 Mount Everest expedition, gave a lecture at the International Design Conference in Aspen, Colorado, about "designing" an expedition. The gist of Beidleman's lecture was that any design—whether for a product, a building, or an expedition—depends on leadership, common group objectives, good equipment, teamwork, and a balance between the flexibility to improvise and a rigid plan to fall back on in the event of a crisis. Beidleman went on to say that the weaknesses in the design of the Everest expedition were exposed by the harsh conditions. What struck me most about Beidleman's lecture was his portrayal of an expedition as a living, breathing entity wherein every part of the design—the equipment, the people, the leadership, and the objectives—all act on each other to form either a successful trip or a failed trip.

Some people seem to have a knack for planning good expeditions. Every year, fellow NOLS instructor and friend Dave Glenn organizes an odd assortment of rednecks, government land managers, and green tree huggers, throws them all together on three or four rubber rafts, floats them through a rough river, and has them finish the adventure making deep political concessions to each other just from the joy of completing a well-designed trip. Dave succeeds at making these impossibly unlikely combinations of people work partly from having a knack with people but also from years of experience, mastery of the planning fundamentals, and surely the experiential benefit of some failures.

In this chapter you will learn a simple outline of variables to consider in designing your own trip. Every trip in the outback involves five main elements: team and leadership; expedition goals; route planning; contingency plans; and ration planning. All these elements, while considered separately for the sake of this chapter, are interconnected and interdependent. The people you bring on your trip will determine the expedition goals; good rations will help keep your group healthy enough to achieve its goals; a well-planned route will help morale. The relationships between these five elements of your plan are endless but the point here is simple: The well-designed trip comes of good planning. Every trip is different, but this outline will help you plan every time.

- ▼ Team and leadership
- ▼ Expedition goals
- ▼ Route planning
- ▼ Contingency plans
- ▼ Ration planning

# Team and Leadership

## IT ALL BEGINS WITH YOU

Before you go, make an honest appraisal of your abilities and experience. This is not the time to pad your résumé, but a time to evaluate your skills, physical condition, and background with some modesty so you will not choose a trip beyond your competence.

Perhaps you are a raw beginner with little or no outdoor experience but a strong athlete and tough as leather. Maybe you have Woody Allen's physique and his affinity for the outdoors as well. Perhaps you have camped a dozen times in the last two years but always with an organized program. Maybe you have a technical background in rock climbing but have never traveled in the Arizona desert, where you are planning to go for your next adventure.

Everyone has certain strengths, be they athletic abilities, mental resilience, or extraordinary patience; and everyone has certain liabilities—fear of heights or poor orientation, for instance. Every year, inexperienced hikers get injured or lost or killed because they attempt trips beyond their abilities. This is not meant to scare you but to raise your awareness. When planning your trip ask yourself these questions:

- ▾ What is the sum total and nature of my outdoor experience?
- ▾ Would I be able to handle an emergency such as a seriously injured or lost party member, or a situation in which I myself was injured?
- ▾ Do I have the physical conditioning and psychological mindset to complete this trip?

## CHOOSING YOUR TEAMMATES

The most important decision you make in planning your trip is who gets to go with you. Your teammates are your best resource in the day-to-day routine and in an emergency. Having good people along—people you enjoy and trust—is the foundation of a good expedition.

After taking stock of your own abilities, consider the abilities and personalities of your teammates. You want a group with matching abilities, compatible personalities, and good judgment. It's certainly fine to bring people of varying skills, but those going should know in advance and agree to be flexible enough to accommodate weaker or less experienced teammates or, when traveling with those who have superior skills, be in a learning role. If you invite a friend with a penchant for long grueling days on the trail, along with a friend who fancies lazy reverie under a banyan tree, you may be asking for a quarrel. Invite a couple intent on consummating their nuptials at every spare moment, and you'll chafe the lone ascetic in the group. Members invited on your trip should know what the pace and style of the trip will be. Perhaps you want to complete a challenging route and do dozens of peak ascents. Perhaps you all just want to get out, relax, fish, and cook lots of good meals. The important thing is that everyone in the group knows what to expect.

If possible, sample your friends on a day hike before you invite them to join you on a long expedition. Even a day of hiking together will give you some idea of their fitness, their attitudes, their moods, and their quirks.

Here are some questions to ask yourself when choosing your teammates:

- ▾ Do they have common sense and good judgment? Would you trust the prospective teammate to get you out of the backcountry if you became incapacitated?
- ▾ Are they of your ability? Will you be comfortable traveling with someone who is much more conservative in judgment than you are, or, conversely, with someone who is much more aggressive?
- ▾ Will you enjoy each other's company?

## GROUP SIZE

Small groups are mobile and involve simple logistics. With a small group you don't have to convene an assembly for every decision about where to hike or what meals to bring. When I go on trips where I want to cover a lot of terrain or climb peaks, I much prefer to travel with a small team. There is less to go wrong and fewer opinions to sway.

Four is often cited at NOLS as a minimum number of people for an expedition. In the event of an injury, one person can stay with the injured party while two people go for help. While traveling in a group of four may be safer than, say, traveling with just one buddy, you should not always feel obligated to travel with three other people. However, you must consider that a smaller group's advantages mean diminished resources (people) in the event of an emergency.

Large groups are raucous good fun but require more formal organization, logistics, and leadership. I love to go on a river trip with four boats and 20 people given one condition: Someone else organizes everything. If the small group can float like a butterfly and sting like a bee, the large group moves like a well-meaning jellyfish.

In a large group you have more personalities, which adds to the fun, but can also slow down the whole decision-making process. Ever try to pick a restaurant with 15 relatives hovering about? With a large group, you have more chances of someone getting injured, simply because of the statistics, but also more resources and options available.

Large groups obviously require more room to camp, and can have a tougher impact on the environment just by sheer volume. If you travel in a large group, you have to work harder to minimize your impact on the environment.

### TRAVELING SOLO

Traveling solo in the backcountry is at once liberating, free, and lonely. The solitude may be just what your soul needs. Alone you will likely see more wildlife, have more flexibility in everything from choosing a campsite to cooking a meal, and perhaps find focus and clarity. But those new to solo travel need to be prepared for the sense of isolation in a vast space. If you travel alone you are in a sense climbing without a rope, and as such, you have less room for error. When traveling solo, you need to be more conservative in nearly everything you do. The river you might cross with a group of friends on hand may be too risky as a lone traveler. An off-trail shortcut you'd take with even one more person might not be wise when alone.

If you do decide to travel solo, learn the art in increments. Start with a single night or two and work your way up to traversing the Pacific Crest Trail. Since you will have no one in the immediate area to watch over you unless there are nearby travelers, you should leave an itinerary with a trusted friend or relative. The itinerary should include the following:

- ▾ A detailed route plan.
- ▾ Where your car will be parked if you drive to the roadhead. Usually the first thing a search and rescue team will check is whether your car is still parked at the roadhead.
- ▾ A generous but well-defined overdue date. If you plan to go for three days, you might tell your contact person you plan to be back on day three but not to send the cavalry until day four or five. The "freak time" should be clearly defined so there is no ambiguity and your friend doesn't call for help either too early or too late.
- ▾ Specific medical problems you have (e.g., diabetes, heart problems, epilepsy, etc.).

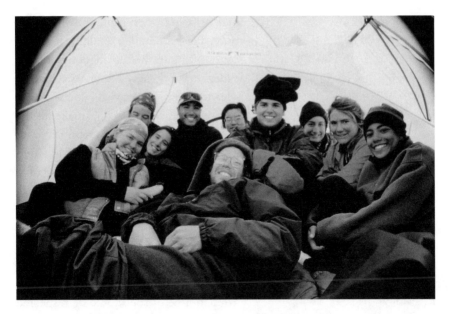

Choosing compatible teammates is one of the important decisions in expedition planning. A NOLS course in the northern Talkeetna Mountains of Alaska. *Fredrik Norrsell*

- ▾ A list of the gear, food, and fuel you are carrying. It is useful for rescue teams to know whether you have a light summer sleeping bag or a heavy bag, a high-quality tent or a sheet of plastic, and food enough for two days or four.
- ▾ Whom to call if you do not arrive on time. Typically this would be the local sheriff or search and rescue team.
- ▾ A description of what you plan to do in an emergency situation (e.g., use a cell phone, a radio, a signal mirror, or a signal fire).

## LEADERSHIP

Chapter 7 discusses leadership in depth, but the matter of leadership and how decisions will be made once out on the trail should be part of your expedition planning. Many people who go out on a trip don't assign formal leadership roles. They make decisions through informal discussions and if there is a leader, he or she arrives at the position through some sort of organic process, not by a conscious and spoken group choice. That style may work well for teams that have traveled together before and have proven to work well together as a team. But when you travel in a large group or when your trip becomes more involved—remote, big mountain expeditions, for instance—you are better off designating a leader. It is arguably better to designate a leader even for trips of small consequence. The leader needn't make all the group's decisions in an autocratic way, but in a crunch, such as a medical emergency, having an official leader could mean faster action. The leader's role may include deciding whether or not to complete a route, planning an evacuation, moderating disputes, and boosting morale. The leader does not necessarily have to be the most experienced in the group, but he or she should be respected by all the members and have excellent judgment.

It may be a little awkward, but if you discuss how day-to-day decisions are going to be made before you leave for the wilds, you will likely have a more successful trip. On all but the most fortunate expeditions, there comes a time when two or more group members don't agree on a matter large or small. If you agree in advance that the person leading that day will resolve the conflict or, on the other hand, that the decision will be made through consensus, you will save yourself the headache of coming up with an ad hoc plan out on the trail.

A trip with every minute and every decision mapped out in advance would be too rigid and would feel like a forced march; some flexibility is necessary to adjust to the mood, health, and desires of the group members. But a leader and a plan should be chosen in advance to deal with the less forgiving circumstances.

## COMMITMENT TO THE TRIP AND THE DIVISION OF LABOR

It is a joy to travel with committed people. Such types troubleshoot sputtering stoves, make coffee on the miserable mornings, and catch meaty trout. Alas, those not committed spend lots of time in the tent (and take up lots of space as well), show pouty faces when the trail gets steep, and have little nice to say about someone's cooking. If you are going to commit good money and dear time to an expedition, better to know your companions feel the same sense of commitment. My friend Phil Powers, a NOLS instructor and highly accomplished mountaineer, suggests assigning planning tasks prior to leaving as a way to test commitment in the group. If, for example, you are traveling to the mountains for four days, have one member organize maps, another rations, and another transportation. If the person responsible for maps doesn't lift a finger as the departure date nears, ask him directly if he wants to go on the trip. Here are a few ways you may want to divide the tasks:

- Ration planning: This person organizes and buys all the food. He or she should poll the other members on likes, dislikes, and allergies. This is a big job so it might take two people.
- Maps, routes, and regulations: This person buys all the maps, researches regulations, and plans the route. As she plans, she can stay in contact with the rest of the group to pose options and solicit ideas.
- Transportation: If your trip is simple—a two-day backpack in the back-yard wilderness—this job may not be necessary. But if you do something exotic, say a trek in Peru, the transportation planning may take phone calls, foreign language skills, trips to the travel agent, and other intricate and time-consuming tasks.
- Equipment planning and revision: This job entails the organization and revision of major group gear including the tent, stove, kitchen utensils, and first aid kit.

## SHARING COSTS

Camping needn't be expensive but there are always costs—gas, food, maps, gear, etc. Find an equitable way to share the costs. If your buddy drives his rig, you pay for the gas. If your buddy brings his new tent, stove, and fishing gear, you spring for the maps. Keep it simple and agree upon it in advance.

## PHYSICAL CONDITIONING

Hiking long miles with a heavy pack is strenuous. Climbing the hills takes strong legs, and balancing the pack weight over tricky stretches on the trail takes a strong back. The men and women who spend their waking hours teaching outdoor education or tackling high mountains fairly ripple with muscle and sinew, the author notwithstanding. All things being equal, the stronger you come into your trip, the more fun you'll have, the more you'll achieve, and the safer you'll be.

A detailed plan is beyond the scope of this book, but the basics are worth mentioning. You don't have to train with the intensity of a marathoner before your trip but try to train for a few weeks prior to leaving. Your regimen should include three components: flexibility training, resistance training, and cardiovascular training.

Developing flexibility before you go will reduce the chances of injury and will add to your agility. Find three or four stretches for the legs, and three or four for the trunk and arms. You can stretch just about anywhere—at the gym, in front of the TV, or at your desk. Out on the trail you may want to do a few stretches every morning as well, especially if you wake up sore and tight.

Resistance training builds muscle mass, which will give you more power and help prevent injuries. You want resistance training that strengthens the entire body. You can do resistance training with weight machines or using your own body weight. Double knee bends (not beyond 90 degrees, please), one-legged knee bends, push-ups, sit-ups, chin-ups, trunk lifts, and weight lifting are all good forms of resistance training.

There are many ways to build your cardiovascular level depending on where you live, your preferences, and how much free time you have. The most obvious and perhaps most logical activity to train for hiking trips is, well, hiking. If you live in a big city, this training may be impossible, but if you have access to the mountains on weekends or during the week, simply get out there and hike the most varied terrain you can find. Walking uphill will build leg strength on top of the cardiovascular conditioning. Walking downhill develops balance and leg strength as well. If you're going to be carrying a heavy pack on your actual trip, you may as well carry a pack in your training. If you are out of shape, start very light—say with ten pounds—and then add five pounds per week until you reach the approximate weight you plan to carry on your trip. Bicycling, running, and swimming are other good forms of exercise for developing your heart and lungs.

# Expedition Goals

## OBJECTIVES AND EXPEDITION PHILOSOPHY

In 1939, seven Americans set out to climb K2, considered by many to be the most difficult mountain in the world.* K2 had never been climbed before. The expedition was led and organized by Fritz Wiessner, a formidable mountaineer already famous for his first ascents on the southeast face of the Fleishbank of the Austrian Tyrol and the north face of the Furchetta in the Dolomites. Wiessner's team consisted of some of the most qualified American mountaineers.

Some two months after the Americans began the climb, three members of the expedition were dead, several others were injured or sick, no one had reached the summit, and certain members of the party parted mortal enemies. It would be unfair to cast harsh judgment on the brave attempt and the competent men who nearly summited K2 in 1939, but we do have the hindsight to see that their disparate expedition objectives and philosophies likely contributed to the harrowing results.

One of the main problems cited by observers among the American alpine community was the difference in climbing philosophy and leadership style between Wiessner and the rest of the team. Wiessner, a German immigrant, ". . . had been reared in the school of absolute obedience to authority that characterizes much of the teutonic ethos: the leader leads and the troops obey, whatever the situation."** His American team, by contrast, was used to more democratic methods of making decisions. As a result, Wiessner did not perfectly understand his team, nor they him. What seemed open communication to the Americans seemed like insubordination to Wiessner. What seemed unreasonably dangerous to the Americans, Wiessner considered a necessary risk in extreme mountaineering.

Ultimately, Wiessner and a teammate named Dudley Wolfe became separated from the rest of the Americans by several camps and several thousand vertical feet. Only Sherpas, who did not speak English, bridged the gap between Wiessner and Wolfe above, and the rest of the team below. Late in the expedition when the team below lost contact with Wiessner for a full eight days, they assumed he had perished. They decided to dismantle the intermediate camps. This would prove fatal for Wolfe and nearly fatal for Wiessner, who later accused the others of attempted murder.

---

*For a good treatment of the 1939 K2 expedition, see Andrew J. Kauffman and William L. Putnam, *K2: The 1939 Tragedy*, Mountaineers Books, 1993.

**K2: The 1939 Tragedy*, p. 33.

One might think that climbing a big mountain like K2 would simply and automatically define the expedition goals. But as the story shows, expedition goals and philosophy can be more subtle and complex. An expedition goal is not just getting from point A to point B or climbing peak X. Expedition goals include where you go but also how you go and even why you go. It's important that everyone on your trip be included in defining the expedition goals. When a person contributes his thoughts and ideas on what direction a trip should take, he will feel more ownership for the outcome and will likely take more responsibility in ensuring that the goals are achieved.

A few years ago, when I climbed Argentina's Aconcagua with a couple of friends, we determined that our expedition goals centered around having some fun, traveling safely, eating well, and maintaining our friendships. Our inventory of gear included ropes and ice axes but also a three-pound spice kit and three books each: The summit was an important goal to us but not at all costs. Our route up Aconcagua was too modest even to be mentioned on the same page as Wiessner's feats, but no matter how modest the route, the three of us left Argentina with a good, worthwhile experience behind us, due in part to our shared objectives and philosophies. Having traveled and worked together before we started the trip, we already knew that our philosophies jibed.

It's quite possible that your gang will start a trip with what you think are common objectives and philosophies, only to discover that you don't see eye to eye. A friend of mine tells the story of a trip she made to the then Soviet Union to do a joint American-Soviet expedition in Kazakhstan. The purpose of the trip was to share scientific expertise, share cultures, and enjoy the mountains. Friction between the two groups developed immediately when members of the American group set out to climb a small peak near the first camp. The Soviets did not like the idea of any travel, no matter how small the trip, without the express permission of the Soviet trip leader. The independent-minded Americans bristled at the infringement on their freedom. Ultimately, the Americans realized that they had to live with the Soviet rules, and the group settled into the business of making a successful expedition.

Common objectives and philosophies do not guarantee a smooth, happy trip. But they certainly increase your odds. It's possible that your group will start with the same objectives but during the trip, time and circumstances will change individuals' aims. When that becomes apparent, it's time to sit down, hash it out, and possibly redefine the what, how, and why of your trip.

## Tips on Planning Your Route

▼ **Mileage** The average back-packer can travel from 5 to 10 miles per day over moderate terrain with a full pack.

▼ **Terrain** The terrain and con-dition of the trails affects your pace. Add about an extra hour to your day for every 1,000 vertical feet you climb.

▼ **First Days Out** Your first days out you will likely be get-ting used to your pack, your boots, and the strenuous exer-cise. If you haven't been out in a while, better to make your first day or two light work.

▼ **Rest Days** On long or stren-uous trips take a rest day every four to six days. Rest days are great opportunities to bake, fish, climb peaks, and just plain rest. Be flexible with your itinerary to take advantage of the best spots or the best times for your breaks.

▼ **Alternatives** When plan-ning your route, look for alter-natives to shorten or lengthen your route. For instance, if you plan a 50-mile loop, there may be a shortcut that knocks off 10 miles should you get behind, or a detour that adds 10 miles if you're feeling particularly strong.

▼ **Avoiding the Crowds** Avoid peak seasons and the most popular trails if you want to get away from it all. Travel midweek if you can. The early fall can also be a great time to avoid crowds.

# Route Planning

## YOUR ROUTE

Good route planning is an art born of lots of experience, a bit of diligence on the planner's part, and a little luck. It's one thing to march from point A to point B on a superhighway trail described in a dozen guidebooks. It's quite another to cre-atively link various river valleys and mountain passes into an interesting loop. If you take the time to study the area you're visiting before your trip, you may avoid unpleasant surprises—trail clo-sures, poor fishing, snowdrifts that stop your horse resupply or your car en route to the trailhead, etc.—and might even learn something that improves your trip.

Once you have chosen the area, find a huge table or a clear floor space, ar-range your maps, and do some finger walking across your route. Every sea-soned camper has calibrated some bodily part to trace distance, whether it's a finger or a few knuckles. Trace out your first day's mileage—whether it's five miles or 15 miles—and see where that puts you for a camp. Is there a water source? Does the terrain look flat enough to camp com-fortably? Where would you camp if you didn't make it to that camp? Taking a mental hike over the maps in front of you, while trying to consider mileage, difficulty of terrain, possible vistas, rest days, fishing holes, shortcuts, evacuation routes, etc., is the best way to plan your route. Bring a fellow traveler in at this stage: Two heads are better than one.

## Regulations That Can Affect Your Trip

▾ Fire: Certain areas become too volatile for fires during droughts.

▾ Group size limit

▾ Bear camping: You may be required to hang your food and practice special bear-camping techniques in areas thick with bears.

▾ Restricted camping areas: Managers restrict areas to protect wildlife or to allow heavily damaged areas to recover.

## REGULATIONS

Nearly all public lands have regulations that will affect your trip. In a dry year, land managers may ban open fires. In heavily used areas, managers may prohibit camping in places with delicate or recovering vegetation. If you're camping in bear country, you may be required to "bear camp" (see Chapter 5) as prescribed by the agency. Many places have restrictions on group size.

The best place to call to get information on these regulations is the local office of the very agency in charge of the land where you plan to travel. If you plan to hike in Colorado National Monument, for instance, call the National Park Service in Fruita, Colorado. If you plan to hike in the Maroon Bells–Snowmass Wilderness Area, call the White River National Forest supervisor.

## MAPS

After deciding where to go, you need to collect all the maps that your route crosses as well as the maps adjacent to your route. We will talk about maps in depth in Chapter 8. Generally the best maps for hiking in the United States are 7.5 minute series United States Geological Survey (USGS) topographical maps. These maps are of such a scale to give you lots of detail on the terrain. The disadvantage of maps of this scale is that you have to spread out several together to get a bigger picture of the whole route. If you're doing a trip of any consequence—let's say more than 50 miles of travel—bring a map that shows the bigger picture as well as 7.5 minute series maps. The USGS and private companies like Trails Illustrated (see sidebar on the following page) make maps drawn to a scale of 1:250,000.

How many sets of maps you bring depends on the number of people in your group, but having two sets makes sense with three or more people. On a rest day, you may decide to climb a peak while your friends descend a valley to go fishing. The extra maps give you the flexibility to do just that. What's more, in the event of an emergency, one set of maps can go with the party going for help while the other set remains with the party that stays with

# Map Sources

## UNITED STATES

▼ **United States Geological Survey (USGS)** The USGS is the nation's largest map source and produces detailed topographical maps of nearly the entire country. This agency is a good starting point for your maps. The USGS also publishes a free "Map Index" for every state.
USGS Information Services
Box 25286
Denver, CO 80225
800-USA-MAPS
Web site: http://mapping.usgs.gov

▼ **National Park Service (NPS)** Maps of all national parks
NPS, Room 1013
Washington, DC 20240
202-208-4747
Web site: http://www.nps.gov

▼ **U.S. Forest Service (USFS)** Maps of all the national forests
USFS, Public Affairs Office, 2nd Floor, Auditor's Building
14th and Independence Avenue S.W., Washington, DC 20250
202-205-1760
Web site: http://www.fs.fed.us

▼ **Trails Illustrated** Maps printed on high quality tearproof, waterproof paper-like plastic. Each map usually covers eight or nine 7.5 minute quadrangles. They make excellent overview maps of your entire route.
Trails Illustrated
P.O. Box 4357
Evergreen, CO 80437
800-962-1643
Web site: http://www.wildfur.com/trails/trailhead.html

▼ **Your Local Camping or Mountaineering Store**

## CANADA

▼ **Canada Map Office** National Topographic Series of maps covers all of Canada's provinces and territories. This agency also has maps of Canada's national parks.
615 Booth Street
Ottawa, Ontario K1A 0E9
613-952-7000

## FOREIGN

▼ **Europe Map Service/OTD Ltd.**
1 Pinewood Road
Hopewell Junction, NY 12533
914-221-0208

▼ **The Map Store**
5821 Karric Square Dr.
Dublin, OH 43017
800-332-7885

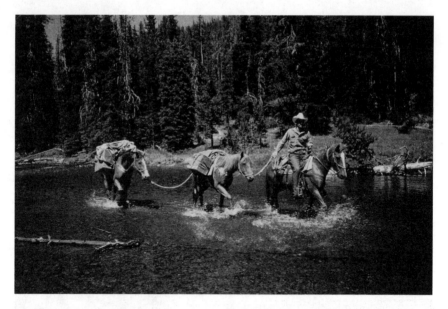

On trips longer than eight or nine days, you'll need a way to resupply your food. Horsepackers are a good option in certain western states because they can bring your rations to you deep in the backcountry. *Mark Harvey*

party going for help while the other set remains with the party that stays with the injured.

## RESUPPLYING YOUR TRIP

If you plan to travel for more than a week, you will probably need to resupply food, fuel, and perhaps first aid supplies. Seven to ten days of food and fuel seems to be the limit for most backs to carry. You can use your resupplies to bring in other things too. For example, you may do a route that involves just hiking on the first half and then rock climbing on the second half. Rather than carry all your climbing gear the entire trip, you can arrange to have it carried in on a resupply.

What means you choose to resupply your trip depends, of course, on where you go. If your trip takes you through areas with accessible roads, you might simply have a friend drive supplies to an agreed-upon trailhead. In Alaska you might need a boat or plane. In Chile, NOLS has even used ox carts.

## Quick and Easy Ways to Resupply Your Trip

▾ Mail your food via general delivery to a post office that intersects or is adjacent to your route. Mark a to-be-picked-up-by date in case you don't make it that far in your trip.

▾ Have a friend meet you at an agreed-upon trailhead.

▾ Make a loop that returns you to your own car or a second car down the trail.

## Resupplying Using Horses

If you're camping in the West, your best bet for a resupply may be with a horse. Horsepackers can handle the oddest loads—from lawn chairs to hay bales—and the sheer size, strength, and agility of a horse gives you the flexibility to haul your food and gear deep into the wilderness. Consult with the packers and they can tell you how they want you to package your supplies. If you have odd-shaped, fragile, or pointy items such as ice axes, photography gear, or weather balloons, tell your packer in advance.

Some horsepackers will buy your fresh produce for you so it doesn't have to sit around wilting for a week. If that's not possible, check to see if they have refrigeration at their barn.

While horses can cross nearly any terrain that a person on foot can handle, keep the following in mind when choosing your resupply site:

▾ Horses have difficulty crossing steep snow slopes or partially melted snowfields. If you are traveling in the late spring or early summer and don't know the snow conditions, either plan your resupply for lower elevations or plan a contingency site in case there is too much snow at the original site.

▾ Your best option may be to let the packer select the resupply site. If he has a regular spot that works with your route, you may save money on the trip. The other advantage to letting the packer choose the site is that he will choose a site that can accommodate his string of horses.

## Resupplying Using Aircraft

In the wilds of Alaska's Brooks Range, British Columbia, or Chile's Patagonia, you may choose a route that has no road crossings or nearby horse ranches. When that's the case, your only option for a resupply may be by plane or helicopter. Remember that in most wilderness areas, using motorized aircraft is illegal except with special permission in emergency evacuations.

A Piper Super Cub airplane costs about $150 per hour, but it can only carry about 200 to 300 pounds, depending on the condition of the airstrip, the weather, and the travel time from the hangar to the ration site.

Helicopters can fly nearly anywhere for a price—yes, for a very hefty price indeed. But if there's no airstrip or the visibility is poor, that may be your only option. Since helicopters can usually handle a bigger payload than a small plane, they are sometimes more cost effective than planes. Helicopters can handle worse weather than their fixed-wing counterparts and land in tighter spots. In short, they are more versatile than fixed-wing airplanes. Depending on the make of the helicopter and the company, you will pay between $400 and $600 per hour.

If you hire a helicopter to do your resupply, keep in mind that the helicopter pilot may choose his landing site only once he sees the area for himself. The site you choose for him may not be the best site so be prepared to move in a hurry.

Regardless of whether you use a helicopter or a fixed-wing plane, the weather will ultimately determine whether or not your pilot can deliver your groceries. Bush pilots have a deserved reputation for their courage in flying in bad weather and in tight spaces. But have a contingency plan in case the weather makes it impossible for your pilot to land. Several friends of mine have waited three days or longer for a break in the Alaska weather so the plane could deliver the groceries.

No matter the method you choose to resupply your trip, you want a site you can comfortably reach on the scheduled day. For instance, if you plan to re-ration on the seventh day of your trip and have scheduled 100 miles of hiking to that site, you might miss your re-ration or run out of food before you get there.

If you do use a third party to resupply your trip and have arranged to meet at an agreed-upon location, be sure to give your resupplier instructions as to where he should leave your supplies if you do not arrive on time.

## USING YOUR COMPUTER
## IN PLANNING YOUR EXPEDITION

If you have a computer, a modem, and Internet access, you can find lots of valuable information to help you plan your route, purchase equipment, and even seek advice on the area where you're going. Several government agencies, equipment manufacturers, and outdoor clubs have helpful Web sites. For instance, the Army Corps of Engineers, the Bureau of Land Management, the Bureau of Reclamation, the Fish and Wildlife Service, the Forest Service, and the National Park Service have joined together to create a site called "Recreation.gov" (http://www.recreation.gov), which offers all sorts of information about specific recreation sites, phone numbers, weather, and overview maps. I live in Colorado so, for the hell of it, I went to the Recreation.gov site and did a search on the Alamosa area. The site offered a description and pictures of the Alamosa National Wildlife Refuge, up-to-the-hour weather information, and several "hyperlinks," which, for those of you new to the Internet, are connections to related sites. One of the hyperlinks for the Alamosa National Wildlife Refuge is the "Avian Page," which lists the bird migration there and tells me that they recently sighted a golden-winged warbler near Alamosa for the first time ever, not to mention three double-crested cormorants!

Another useful site is the one maintained by the National Weather Service (http://iwin.nws.noaa.gov), which offers local, national, and international forecasts. They of course have hyperlinks, one of which is a weather glossary. Did you know that the word "scud" means "small, ragged, low cloud fragments that are unattached to a larger cloud base and are often seen with and behind cold fronts and thunderstorm gust fronts"? You'll find that term and others on the National Weather Service weather glossary.

If you wanted to hike the Pacific Crest Trail and needed a partner to do it, you could check out http://saffron.hack.net/lists/, a Web page dedicated to national scenic trails. On that page, I found people looking for partners to do various sections of the trail, tips on equipment, route suggestions—if the Baden-Powell section is too snowy, take the Manzanita Trail—and querulous essays disparaging certain government agencies managing sections of the Pacific Crest Trail.

If you're interested in taking a NOLS course, visit the NOLS Web site at http://www.nols.edu. The site lists dates and descriptions of the various NOLS courses, a list of NOLS publications, and information on how to contact the school.

There are millions of Web pages on the Internet, some of them extremely useful, some perfectly useless, and some merely amusing. But if you learn to focus your searches with Boolean commands (talk to your computer geek friend about that), you can use your computer and modem as a powerful tool to plan your expedition.

# Contingency Plans

When NASA planned the Apollo missions to the moon in the sixties, they had to make contingency plans based on the unknown. No one had ever landed a spaceship on another planet and there was no way of knowing for sure what might go wrong. All the scientists could do was imagine what might fail and plan backup systems based on their educated guesses. Drawing a parallel between your trip to the backcountry and a trip to the moon may be labored, but there are some useful analogies. When you go to the backcountry, you leave a very organized system that you know backward and forward for a system with less infrastructure and more of the unfamiliar. You can make educated guesses about what might go wrong in the wilds, but there are many unknowns, which you simply can't anticipate with any consistency, especially if you're going to a new area. But that's no reason to throw your hands up in despair and say, "We'll just deal with the problems when they arise." You can make sound contingency plans for your expedition by considering both the typical ways in which people get in trouble in the backcountry and the particular vulnerabilities of your group.

Contingency planning is an exercise in imagining the unimaginable. You can start by asking yourself what you would do if one of your party members became sick or injured. Types of injuries you might expect in the outdoors include sprains, broken bones, dislocations, lacerations, frostbite, hypothermia, and hyperthermia. Illnesses include gastrointestinal sickness caused by bacteria or viruses as well as diseases caused by bites or stings from local fauna. It is unlikely that someone on your trip through the Green Mountains of Vermont will break his femur, but it's not impossible. It is unlikely that someone on your trip to the mountains of Baja California will get bit by a rattlesnake, but also not impossible. To be prepared for contingencies, then, you should know at least rudimentary, and, preferably, advanced first aid.

A good contingency plan also calls for knowing when and how to evacuate a person in the event of a serious injury or illness and what outside assistance is available. These skills require training not just in first aid, but in *wilderness* first aid. Understanding the communication systems in the area where you take your trip is also an important element in a contingency plan. By communication systems, I mean everything from trails, roads, and locations of pay phones that can be used by an evacuation team, to electronic devices such as cell phones and radios. When you spread out your maps to plan your route, take note of the surrounding areas, geographical features, roads, and townships. You may plan a simple route that takes you up to a lake and back over a period of five days. Were someone to be seriously injured at the lake, the shortest route for help might be in the opposite direction from where you came. Perhaps you see the symbol for a building on your map fewer than five miles from the lake. In your planning it's worth finding out if that building is the remains of a ghost town or an active ranch. Making a few phone calls to land management agencies, the local sheriff, search and rescue groups, outfitters, and local clubs and talking to local sports shops can really help you to understand the available communication systems and thereby make a better contingency plan. It's worth bringing along the maps that show you alternative routes out of the backcountry.

## RADIOS, CELL PHONES, AND OTHER ELECTRONIC COMMUNICATION DEVICES

Radios, cell phones, and other electronic communication devices can be very useful in the case of emergencies. NOLS courses around the world utilize a wide variety of electronic communication devices, including many different types of radios and cell phones. If you wish to use these tools, it is important to understand their limitations, which may include weight, expense, range, battery life, licensing regulations, and durability. The danger with carrying a phone or a radio is that it can give people a false sense of security and cause them to forget the remote setting and the complicated logistics of an evacuation. Climbers and backpackers armed with cell phones have called mountain shops for directions from the backcountry. Parties have called 911 for help with problems that they obviously should have been prepared for. In these cases, the phones and radios acted as a crutch that kept the parties from relying on themselves and planning their expeditions with more care. If you do carry a radio, it's important that you not let it prevent you from being self-sufficient and safe.

Don't assume that your cell phone or radio will work everywhere in the world. Remember that to make a connection with a cell phone you need to be within range of a "cell site" and there are lots of "holes" over the wilderness areas. If you bring a ground-to-air radio to a place where there are no overhead flights—parts of Alaska, for instance—it will be no more useful than trying to communicate with your hands cupped around your mouth and bellowing for help.

The choice of whether to bring a radio or not is a personal one. If you are traveling with a large group in an institutional setting, the argument for bringing a radio is strong—even if only for liability concerns. In small private groups, a radio may help cut a day off an evacuation. If you decide to carry a radio, know how to use it, when to use it, and its limitations.

# Ration Planning

The only thing certain in ration planning is that if you don't bring enough food, you'll likely find yourself eating something disgusting when the rations run out. NOLS instructor Andy Cline tells of the time he ran out of food deep in the southern Andes on a month-long hiking trip. He and his friends had the good fortune to find a remote farm and a farmer willing to sell them a lamb. They lived off the best parts of the lamb for a few days—the loins and the ribs—but soon they were into the less appealing parts—the brains, in-testines, liver, and gonads. Competent mountaineers all, but sorely lacking in the study of nutrition, they devoured the liver with the result that their skins turned a ghastly orange from the near-toxic concentrations of vitamin A. Fi-nally, they made brain soup. If the story has no moral instruction, it is never-theless scientific proof that eating the brains of another animal does very little to improve the human intellect.

The movies always depict the lost traveler eating rich meals off the land—pheasant eggs, fresh salmon, ripe blackberries—when they run out of food, but unless you've really learned how to scavenge, you'll go hungry.

## STAPLE FOOD VERSUS FREEZE-DRIED FOOD

When you plan your rations for the outdoors, you can either take staples such as pasta, flour, dried beans, rice, sugar, etc., or you can take specially pre-pared camping food like freeze-dried meals or boil packets. In general, we recommend staple food for a few reasons:

- ▾ It's much cheaper. A freeze-dried dinner listed as a meal for two costs be-tween five and seven dollars. In my experience these meals really feed only one person. And for that money, you could easily pay for an entire day's worth of staple food.
- ▾ It's easier to find. Whether you're traveling in the United States or in Bo-livia, it's easier to find something like pasta or potatoes than it is to find high-quality freeze-dried food.
- ▾ It allows you more flexibility. With staple food you can mix and match ingredients to your heart's desire and, with a little effort, cook delicious meals. With prepackaged food, you are limited to the company's choice of meals—a sort of carte fixe.

Let's not dismiss freeze-dried meals out of hand. The truth is freeze-dried meals have their place in your quiver of tricks. They weigh less than staple food. If you need to travel great distances and can't arrange a resupply or cache, you can carry freeze-dried meals. What's more, they are convenient. To prepare most freeze-dried meals, you simply add hot water. On demanding routes, easy-to-prepare meals make it that much easier to concentrate on the tasks at hand. If you're climbing a major mountain, for instance, you may not want to think about cooking. You may have enough to concentrate on with the weather, the altitude, and the long days. Perhaps you're not the type who likes to cook. Perhaps you're eighty years old and limited to a small pack weight. What's more, some companies have developed tasty freeze-dried meals.

## TYPES OF STAPLE FOODS

### Trail Foods

**Nuts and Seeds.** Nuts such as peanuts, almonds, cashews, Brazil nuts, and walnuts, and seeds such as sunflower seeds and sesame seeds are high in energy, fat, and protein, make good trail food, and add nice texture and flavor to things like pancakes, dinner dishes, and breads. Buy the shelled nuts so you don't have to pack out more garbage.

**Dried Fruit.** Dried peaches, apples, apricots, plums, pineapples, and raisins are high in carbohydrates and fiber. They make a good snack but can also be soaked in warm water and rehydrated to use in dessert dishes such as cobblers or dinner dishes such as curries. The sulphured fruits last longer than the fruits processed naturally.

**Energy Bars and Fruit Bars.** Several companies such as Power Bar and Cliff Bar make high-energy snacks loaded with complex carbohydrates, vitamins, and minerals. They're expensive but simple snacks that give a great deal of energy. Drink lots of water with these so they digest properly. Halvah bars and pemmican bars are other good options for high-energy blasts.

**Breadstuffs.** On short trips or if eaten early on long trips, it's nice to bring hearty breads such as bagels or pita bread. They go well with cheese or peanut butter, can be fried with cheese for a breakfast, or eaten as a side with dinner. Bagels and pita bread will withstand the rigors of backpacking better than regular bread. Rye crisp, melba toasts, bagel chips, pretzels, zwiebacks, and the like are also durable and good with cheese.

**Trail Mixes.** You can buy or make your own trail mixes from a wide variety of snacks. Try nuts, raisins, M&Ms, dried fruit, crackers, banana chips, and whatever else suits your fancy.

**Jerky and Salami.** I like to make my own elk and beef jerky for the trail. It's a nice source of protein and, if prepared properly, will last on long trips. See Chapter 11 for how to make jerky. Salami lasts several days on the trail, though you should try to keep it cool.

**Fruit Leathers.** You can buy fruit leather commercially or make your own using a dehydrator. High in energy, it's a good alternative to sweets.

### Dinner Foods

**Pasta.** Pasta is rich in complex carbohydrates, easy to prepare, can be made into any one of several delicious dishes, is inexpensive, travels well, and is almost universally liked. In short, it's one of the best dinner staples you can bring—the uber-food. If you're going on a long trip, bring a variety of styles—spaghetti, macaroni, and penne—and a few flavors—white, wheat, and spinach. Pasta makes a good breakfast too.

**Rice.** Like pasta, rice can be used as the base of several recipes. It's a good source of carbohydrates and, prepared with beans, makes a complete protein. Except for the instant variety, rice takes longer to cook than pasta.

**Other Grains.** Couscous, a Middle Eastern staple food, cooks quickly and can be prepared with some of the same recipes you use to prepare pasta. Cooked with brown sugar and cinnamon, it makes a nice breakfast. Bulgur is a wheat product with a lot of fiber and texture. Use it in place of rice for some variety. Falafel, another Middle Eastern food, is made from ground chick-peas, yellow split peas, and lots of spices. It can be made into patties and fried for a savory dinner.

**Legumes.** Beans are the basis for lots of Mexican recipes, go well with rice, and are easy to cook. Bring the quick-cooking beans unless you have a pressure cooker or are willing to take the trouble to soak them. Lentils make nice soups but need soaking and lots of time to cook.

**Potatoes.** There are a few forms of dried potatoes: flakes, pearls, and dehydrated hash browns. With the flakes and pearls you can make an instant meal simply by adding hot water and something like a powdered soup base to flavor it. At the end of a hard day when you don't have energy to cook, potato pearls and flakes may be just what you need for dinner. The dehydrated hash browns take a little longer to cook but can be enjoyed for breakfast or dinner.

**Cheese.** Cheese, if not left out in the sun too often, lasts a surprisingly long time out on a camping trip. Low-fat and hard cheeses last even longer. It is good for pizza, Mexican meals, breads, and more. It also makes a nice snack on the trail. Cheese is high in protein and fat.

**Meats.** If your packs aren't too heavy, bring along a can of chicken or tuna as a nice addition to pasta, rice, bulgur, beans, or couscous. Once opened, however, the meat should be consumed immediately so you don't have problems with food-borne illnesses.

**Soups and Bases.** Miso, ramen, powdered soups, and bouillon don't weigh much, and are inexpensive and very nice on a cold evening. They also make easy bases for sauces or good flavorings for a main dish. If someone on the trip has an upset stomach from the altitude or bacteria, a simple soup may be the best solution.

### Breakfast Foods

**Cold cereals** like granola, Grape-Nuts, and Cracklin' Oat Bran can be eaten for a quick breakfast or as a snack out on the trail.

**Hot Cereals.** Oatmeal, cream of wheat, and seven-grain cereals define the word hearty. They make a good breakfast for a long day and are simple to prepare. Buy the instant versions so you don't have to spend too much time cooking in the morning. You can add rehydrated dried fruit, nuts, cinnamon, and brown sugar to make these cereals a little more interesting.

**Pancakes.** If you have a little extra time—perhaps on a rest day—and plenty of stove fuel, pancakes add a certain civility to any outdoor breakfast. You can buy the ready-to-cook mixes, or make your own from flour, baking powder, milk, and salt. Make your syrup with a little melted butter and some brown sugar.

### Baking Materials

Flour, both white and whole wheat, can be used to make bread, pancakes, pizza crusts, and cinnamon rolls. White flour is good for making gravy or white sauces, as well as for dredging your trout.

Cornmeal is, of course, the base for corn bread, but also for tortillas, chapatis, and the hot cereal, polenta. Fresh trout dredged in cornmeal, salt, and pepper, then fried in margarine is delicious.

Baking mix, such as Bisquick or your own homemade version, simplifies making pancakes, pizza crusts, and biscuits.

### Beverages

Fruit crystals (good for flavoring water)

Coffee and tea

Instant cocoa

Apple cider mix

Powdered milk for cold cereals, baking, casseroles, or for a warm mug of milk before bed

## A Word on Fresh Foods

Unless you have a good way to keep your food cool (below 40° F), bringing along fresh foods such as meat, poultry, fish, and dairy products is a bad idea because of the danger of spoilage. These types of fresh foods, if not stored properly, make perfect breeding grounds for wretched bacteria such as campylobacter and salmonella, which can make you seriously ill. But if weight is not an issue, it's nice to bring an onion, a few potatoes, or some other hardy vegetable that doesn't spoil easily.

## Herbs and Spices

Bringing along a few herbs and spices and knowing how to use them is the basis for good backcountry cooking. Finding the right combination and the right proportions of herbs and spices comes with brave experimentation and close study of the master chefs in your expedition. Begin by mastering a few simple combinations such as oregano, garlic, and basil. Here is a list of versatile herbs and spices for your trip. Pick and choose the ones that suit your fancy.

- ▼ Basil is a green, leafy herb (green flakes in its dried form) that smells somewhat like licorice and mint. It goes well with tomato sauces, Italian dishes, and any kind of fresh trout.
- ▼ Black pepper is the most versatile of the spices (in the Middle Ages, a pound of black pepper would buy a serf's freedom) and can be put in any dish to pep it up. Some people even put a pinch of pepper in a fruit cobbler to bring out the cinnamon. For the brave ones, put a tiny bit in your hot chocolate. You'll be surprised.
- ▼ Cayenne powder, which looks like paprika, is made from the thin red peppers and is very hot—between 30,000 and 50,000 Scoville heat units (the Scoville system is a way for pepper growers to measure how hot chili peppers are; the banana pepper is rated at 0 Scoville units and the habañero is rated at 300,000 units). It only takes a pinch.
- ▼ Cinnamon (made from the bark of the evergreen laurel tree) is brilliant in sweet rolls, pancakes, cobblers, Mexican dishes, curries, hot cider, and tea.
- ▼ Cumin has a pungent, smoky flavor and goes well with curry, cinnamon, and cayenne. It is the basis for many Mexican dishes and a good addition to rice and soups. Cumin is also nice in corn bread. A little goes a long way.
- ▼ Curry is an Indian spice (actually made from a combination of as many as 20 different spices) with a bright yellow color. Curry dishes can be

made with rice, bulgur, lentils, and soups. Hot peppers and dried fruit such as raisins or apricots go well with curry.

▼ Dill is a member of the same family that includes caraway, cumin, and coriander. The name dill comes from the Norse word *dilla,* which means to lull. Dill does indeed have a mild sedative effect. Dill goes well in breads, with fish, pasta, and soups. The more you cook dill, the less flavor it has, so add it toward the end.

▼ Garlic comes in powder, flakes, and of course in fresh cloves. This herb makes an Italian dish Italian or a Mexican dish Mexican. Fresh garlic in the backcountry adds a refined touch to your meals. Simmer it in oil to bring out the flavor.

▼ Mustard can be hydrated and used in salad dressings for the fresh greens you pick along the trail, with casseroles, beans, or pasta. If the mustard is too strong for your taste, try hydrating it with a little vinegar for a milder mix.

▼ Salt. If your meal tastes flat, it is probably lacking in salt, the Viagra of spices.

▼ Soy sauce, a salty product of fermented soybeans, goes well with rice dishes, pasta, and soups.

▼ Vanilla, a member of the orchid family, was used by the Aztec Indians to flavor their chocolate. Vanilla is still good in hot chocolate, pancakes, puddings, and dessert cakes.

▼ Vinegar adds a pungent taste to sweet and sour dishes and makes a nice salad dressing (with some oil).

## BRINGING THE RIGHT AMOUNT OF FOOD

It's not easy to hit your food quantities dead on for long trips in the mountains, but unfortunately you don't have a lot of room for error. If you bring too much, you have to hump a huge pack up the trail. If you don't bring enough you may find yourself eating sheep brains. Our discussion here deals with staple food, not freeze-dried meals.

Over the years, the better minds who plan rations at NOLS have learned that the average person eats between 1.5 and 2.5 pounds of food per person per day out in the mountains, or between 2,500 and 4,500 calories. There is a 60 percent difference between 1.5 pounds and 2.5 pounds so the weights bear discussion. Consider what sort of eaters you have in your group. An adolescent requires near hourly feeding. Some people eat lightly regardless of size, while others seem to consume their body weight in food. If you're camping with new people, be wary of those who say, "Don't bring much for me, I eat like a bird." Perhaps they eat like a bird in the city but out in the hills, humping their pack over the miles, they probably eat like a ravenous emu. Besides, some birds eat their body weight in food every day.

How much food you eat also depends on how strenuous a trip you plan. You'll eat less food while hiking light days in the summer than you will ski mountaineering in January. You'll eat more food on a climbing trip than you will on a fishing trip. The table below can help you to decide how much food to ration.

If you're going for a short trip of five days or less, it's easiest to just plan your ration meal by meal. Once you have put together your menu for the trip, it's a good idea to weigh all the food and divide the total poundage by the total number of person-days to make sure your quantities are within reason. For instance, on a five-day trip with four people, you have a total of 20 person-days. If your crew is going on a typical backpacking trip, based on the table below, you would want to bring between 30 and 40 pounds of staple food. If your total poundage is over or under that number, you know you need to rethink your menu.

On longer trips, it may be too complicated to plan out every single meal. Claudia Pearson, author of *NOLS Cookery* and rations manager at the NOLS Rocky Mountain branch, plans rations for literally thousands of people per year. She does her planning by calculating the number of person-days, multiplying that number by the pounds per day (1.5–2.5 pounds), and then breaking down that number into specific food groups based on the pie chart on page 60. For instance, 4 people traveling for 10 days would need 80 pounds of food (assuming they decide to bring 2 pounds per person per day). Based on the pie chart, their menu would include 12.8 pounds of breakfast food, 17 pounds of trail food, 14.4 pounds of dinner food, 10.1 pounds of cheese, 5.33 pounds of sugar and fruit drinks, 5.9 pounds of flour and baking mix, 3.2

*Figure 2-1 Ration Table\**

| | Average Wilderness Activities (Backpacking or Kayaking) | Strenuous Wilderness Activities (Snowcamping) | Very Strenuous Activities (Extreme Mountaineering) |
|---|---|---|---|
| **Pounds per person per day** | 1.5–2 | 2–2.25 | 2.25–2.5 |
| **Calories per person per day** | 2,500–3,000 | 3,000–3,700 | 3,700–4,500 |

*Source: *NOLS Cookery*

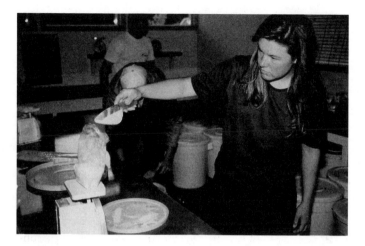

Weighing staples. On long expeditions getting the ration weights just right keeps the group well fed without being overburdened by extra weight. NOLS groups use food scales to make sure they bring the right amount of staple food. *Theo Singelis*

pounds of soups, bases, and desserts, and 11.2 pounds of milk, eggs, margarine, and cocoa.

Rarely do you bring just the right amount of food. Chances are, you'll come back with a little extra food, which isn't a bad thing. You won't have a refined sense of ration planning until you get some experience with it. If you camp often, you should make some notes on how much food you bring each trip and how that food fared. Did you stuff yourself every day and still come back with 10 pounds of extra food? Next time lop a few points off your equation. Did you finish your ration two days before the end of your trip and spend the last twenty miles on a spiritual fast that you neither wanted nor enjoyed? Next time jack up your ration calculation. Did you arrive at the roadhead with but one dried apple in your pack, content and well fed? Bravo!

## PACKAGING YOUR FOOD

There's no sense bringing all the paper, cardboard, and plastic packaging that most foods come in—it's extra weight and often ends up as backcountry litter—so once you've bought all your rations, it's best to repackage it in two-ply plastic bags. If you bring something that has special instructions for its preparation, clip it out and put it in the plastic bag. Be sure your plastic bags are of at least two-ply strength or you'll likely have powdered milk or some such spill all over your belongings. Tie the bags with a *loose* overhand knot (who wants to fiddle with a tightly clenched knot on a cold day?) and, if you

*Figure 2-2 Staple Food Pie Chart*

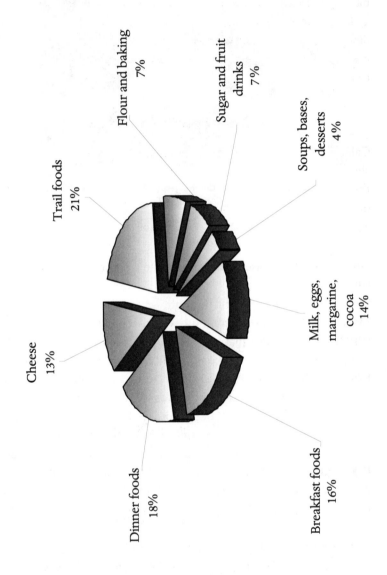

like, mark the difficult-to-identify ingredients with an indelible marker to identify the contents. For liquids like soy sauce, cooking oil, and vinegar, the plastic nalgene bottles with the screw-tops work well. The wide-mouthed nalgene tubs are best for things like peanut butter and margarine.

Finally, let me give you one of NOLS's best trade secrets—nylon zip bags. Since you have to get at your food every day, you want a bag that gives you easy access. Nylon zip bags allow you to see and get at your victuals with ease.

## FUEL CALCULATIONS

Calculate the quantity of fuel to bring as part of your ration planning. You should check the stove manufacturers' recommendations, but, typically, three people using one camp stove in the summer will burn about half a quart of fuel per day. Put another way, you should ration about one-sixth of a quart of fuel per person per day for summer trips.

That equation changes dramatically if you plan to camp on a glacier for your entire trip. In that scenario, you will need to melt liters and liters of snow for both cooking and drinking. You might have your stove running for two hours in the morning and two hours at night just melting snow. Double the fuel ration to about one-third of a quart of fuel per person per day for trips that require melting snow for water.

If you like to bake or if you drink lots of hot drinks, tea and the like, you need to bring extra fuel too. Baking, especially, can drain a fuel bottle quickly.

# Summary for Your Expedition Planning

If you assess your own abilities, choose your teammates well, define the objectives of your trip, study and plan your route, calculate rations and fuel, and get yourself into good physical shape, you have prepared well for your trip.

- ▼ **Team and Leadership.** Assess yourself and your teammates. Put together a group of people you trust. Aim for a group that wants to achieve the same goals on the trip. Choose a person with excellent judgment who is respected by the whole group to be your leader.
- ▼ **Expedition Goals.** Discuss the goals of the trip with your teammates before you go. Discuss the what, where, why, and how. If objectives change during the trip, sit down and discuss new objectives.

▾ **Route Planning.** Study your route and discuss it with your teammates over a full set of maps. Learn the regulations where you will be traveling. For longer trips, decide on the best form of resupply given the remoteness of the area you're traveling in, and then select the best site with the pilot, horsepacker, or friend who will do the resupply.

▾ **Contingency Plans.** Try to imagine the unimaginable before you go and then ask yourself how you would manage an emergency situation. Learn the communication systems—trails, roads, and nearby phones—of the area.

▾ **Ration Planning.** Staples are less expensive than freeze-dried foods and allow more flexibility and creativity in your meals. Freeze-dried foods are lighter than staple foods and easier to prepare. Bring freeze-dried foods if you need to go super-light or need the convenience. On short trips, you can plan your rations on a per-meal basis. On long trips, it's easier to ration between 1.5 and 2.5 pounds per person per day, depending on the difficulty of your route and the nature of travel.

# CHAPTER 3

# Equipment Primer

Then came the gadgeteer, otherwise known as the sporting-goods dealer. He has draped the American outdoorsman with an infinity of contraptions, all offered as aids to self-reliance, hardihood, woodcraft, or marksmanship, but too often functioning as substitutes for them. Gadgets fill the pockets, they dangle from neck and belt. The overflow fills the auto-trunk and also the trailer. Each item of outdoor equipment grows lighter and often better, but the aggregate poundage becomes tonnage.

—Aldo Leopold, *A Sand County Almanac*

I have seen complex personality changes, dilated eyes, and intensely focused expressions among friends and acquaintances entering one of those well lit, tastefully decorated outdoor sports stores. I admit that my pulse races a bit and I feel somewhat faint when I enter a store lined with rows and rows of colorful, high-tech equipment. It's a dangerous thing to go into one of these places with freshly minted money or good credit and an appetite for the best gear. But I would boil it down to this: look for good gear, not fancy gear.

One thing I've noticed about the outdoorspeople I most admire is that they pack small sleek packs, and yet they always seem to have enough gear to stay warm and dry, catch fish, take photos, and cook good meals. They are disciplined in what they bring and what they leave at home. Over the years they have tried enough different gear to be discriminating, even skeptical in what they buy. In my conversations with seasoned NOLS instructors and other accomplished outdoorspeople, I've noticed a common thread with regard to outdoor equipment: Yes, they appreciate and depend on good materials, technology and gear. But they are generally skeptical about "The Tent" or "The Stove" or "The Pack." Most are gadget-shy.

In an effort to outsell competitors, some outdoor equipment manufacturers have festooned their gear with zippers, pockets, extra blades, snaps, Velcro, hinges, and the like. Reading the promotional literature, I have often been convinced that I will actually become a better human being if I just buy that one piece of gear.

I do not want to disparage equipment designers. The good ones have truly made our lives easier in the outdoors with a tent that can face a stiff wind, a stove that roars with heat, or a sleeping bag so filled with ethereal goose down that it can only be described as voluptuous. And most gear today is lighter and stronger than gear of ten years ago.

Nor do I want to give you the impression that finding equipment of high quality is not important. If you plan to do a trip of any consequence, certain of your gear should be selected very carefully, and the extra time and/or money should be spent to buy something of high quality. Take your tent, for instance. In a raging storm, your happiness and comfort—if not your life— depend on your tent, and don't count on constructing a makeshift shelter out of pine boughs if your $50 plastic tube tent gets torn asunder by the wind. Sure, in an emergency you can fashion a shelter from something in the woods, but it won't give the same protection and comfort of a good commercially made tent or fly and the consequences will jeopardize your expedition. With things you count on day in and day out for shelter, protection,

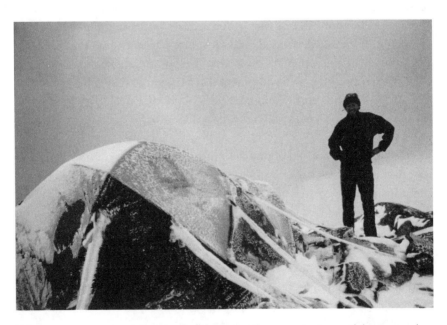

When it comes to a crucial piece of equipment such as your tent, spend the time and money to find something of high quality. Imagine spending a rime-frosted night like this in a flimsy tent. *Andy Tyson*

traveling, and emergencies—things like your sleeping bag, footwear, tent, and stove—you want to make sure you have high-quality gear that's in good condition.

Otherwise, the small things—trying to save money on a crucial piece of equipment, or missing a step on an equipment checklist—can stop an expedition dead in its tracks. Sue Giller, a very accomplished mountaineer with seven major Himalayan expeditions to her credit, tells the story of the time her team's efforts to save $500 on stoves ended up costing the expedition $5,000, a week's delay, and nearly the successful completion of the trip. In 1992, Giller's team planned to cross the Greenland ice cap on skis to train for an all-women's trans-Antarctic expedition scheduled for later that same year.

Giller was in charge of equipment for the Greenland trip and tried in vain to get sponsorship from a major camp stove company. Strapped for funds, Giller and company didn't want to shell out $500 to purchase new stoves and after some phone calls finally found someone willing to loan them some. While still in the United States, Giller checked the stoves and noticed they did not have universal burners and were set up to burn only white gas. Giller called her contacts in Greenland to make sure that white gas was readily available and was assured that indeed it was. The team flew to Greenland, purchased what they thought was white gas, and then flew by helicopter out to the ice cap. After the helicopter had left, Giller's team set up camp, and tried to light up their stoves. To their dismay, they realized that what was supposed to be white gas was actually pure aviation kerosene and despite trying several tricks, the stoves would not burn without getting gummed up immediately. The expedition made faint radio contact with the helicopter base and was able to communicate—just barely—their location and the problem with the stoves. Nearly a week later, the helicopter flew new stoves and new fuel to the expedition—at a cost of $5,000. To confound things, the delay meant that the team had to stretch 32 days' worth of food over 41 days.

When I asked Giller if the story had a moral, she replied, "If you're planning a big trip, you've got to pay attention to details. Don't skimp on the three most important pieces of equipment: your tent, your stove, and your footwear. Make a planning checklist and then follow it point by point. We meant to check the stove-fuel combination in Greenland but got rushed and missed that step. It cost us $5,000 and nearly the trip."

It might help you to think of your equipment choices in utilitarian terms. When you go on a camping trip, you need equipment that will allow you to stay warm and dry, sleep comfortably, eat well, travel (whether on foot, boat, or horse), and deal with a medical emergency. The equipment that allows you to accomplish these things safely and efficiently is the right choice of equipment—period.

## Where to Buy Your Equipment

There are several advantages to buying your gear in person rather than by mail order. If it's an item that needs to be fitted—boots, for instance—shopping in person will give you a chance to compare several different sizes. When you go to the store itself, you can see, touch, squeeze, smell, or even lick the product to decide if it's the best item for your money. It's comforting to see what you are purchasing in real life before you buy it and you might even learn something important inspecting it closely. If you're buying a piece of equipment that you don't know enough about to make an informed decision, a good salesperson can guide you to making a better purchase. My experience with salespeople in outdoor stores has generally been positive. Many are simply rock-climbing addicts or kayakers trying to support a habit with a day job. Find the right one and he or she will provide you with more information than you ever asked for. Finally, outdoor stores often share good information about surrounding areas, be it fishing tips or climbing sites, and by shopping locally you do your little part to ensure their survival.

If your local store doesn't have a wide selection of gear, its prices are outrageously high, or if your local outdoor store simply doesn't exist, you will want to mail-order your gear. There are some huge camping retailers that offer good prices. If you plan to buy a lot of gear, consider joining a cooperative like Recreational Equipment Incorporated (REI). With each purchase you earn credit toward an end-of-the-year dividend. The dividends vary, but in 1996, REI paid its members dividends of 10 percent of their purchases. Campmor and Eastern Mountain Sports are two other big, reputable camping retailers. The best outdoor equipment manufacturers have good catalogs that explain materials, features, and the function of their product.

Another option, if you have a computer and modem, is to buy your gear on the Internet. Several suppliers have set up Web sites that allow you to browse virtually and then make your purchase with a credit card and a few clicks of the mouse. Some of the Web sites I've explored are educational and teach you about materials, weights, sizes, and shapes, in addition to having photos of the items.

Consider buying used gear, too. Some camping stores have bulletin boards with lots of used goods advertised. If you live in an active sports town, you may even see bulletin boards with used camping gear at the grocery store.

There is not enough space in this book to evaluate every model and brand out there, so if you want specifics on gear features, prices, and even ratings, I recommend the annual "Gear Guide" published by *Backpacker* magazine or the "Buyers' Guide" published by *Outside* magazine.

# Footwear

Your footwear is arguably the most important part of your gear, especially if you are planning to hike long days or climb difficult peaks. Invest the time and money to select and buy good boots and you will be infinitely more happy in the mountains than your counterparts who hastily buy bargain shoes. Cowboys have an old saying: "No hoof, no horse." If you're going backpacking, take that same advice: No hoof, no hiker. Poorly fitted boots or boots of low quality will leave your feet an ugly mess of blisters. In the mountains, where it is not easy to keep your feet dry and clean, blisters take a long time to heal and rubbing your feet raw may mean you have to shorten your trip to wait for your feet to heal. What's worse, open blisters can lead to infection.

## BOOT SELECTION

Boots have become lighter and more comfortable over the last ten years. Older boots were put together with what's known in the trade as a "Norwegian welt," wherein the upper was stitched to the midsole. New adhesives allow manufacturers to cement the upper to the midsole, making the boots less expensive, lighter, more comfortable, and easier to break in. The mid soles of yesteryear's boots were simply layers of leather surrounding a steel shank. With the old construction, boot designers were not able to micro-adjust the boot's flex to match the size of the boot. Small people suffered breaking in their boots since a size six boot had the same flex as a size twelve boot. New shanks are made of nylon and the resulting flex makes for a more comfortable boot and a gentler break-in period. What's more, they're warmer. Boot designers have also incorporated molded foot beds and plastic heel cups to give you a much better fit than boots of yesteryear.

The inside of today's boots are often lined with wicking material that makes the boot dry faster. More expensive boots will even have a Gore-Tex liner to allow breathability and still keep your foot dry. On the top of the modern boot, you'll notice that designers have put in a groove to accommodate your Achilles tendon and a padded collar to keep debris out. The new soles have a tapered lug pattern that is said to shed mud more easily.

Your selection of boots will depend on the terrain you plan to cross, the weight you carry, and the climate, but also on personal preference. The truth of the matter is that some people like a very lightweight boot for the task at hand (see the John Roskelley interview on page 91), while others like a heavy boot even on moderate terrain. On most NOLS wilderness courses, students and instructors wear what's known as a rough trail boot. The boot offers good ankle support, an aggressive sole, a degree of water resistance, and is not too heavy. This boot is a good selection if you're carrying a big pack (say 40 percent of your body weight) and crossing difficult terrain. Once worn out, the molded soles of these boots can be replaced for about $40 to $60.

If you're just going out for a weekend trip, you can step down a grade in boots to what's known in the trade as the off-trail boot. The off-trail boot is lighter and more flexible than the rough trail boot, but still offers above-the-ankle support, full-grain leather uppers, and an aggressive sole. These boots take less time to break in than the rough trail boot, but they aren't as durable.

Still lighter weight and more flexible are the trail boots or light hikers. These boots are usually constructed of fabric and leather. They are heavier and more sturdy than tennis shoes but lighter than off-trail boots. They have a flexible sole and should feel comfortable right out of the store (i.e., they don't need to be broken in). These boots are fine for day hikes or overnight trips with a light pack, but if you are carrying a pack of more than 20 pounds, consider moving up into a sturdy boot. Light hikers make nice camp shoes, too, because they offer enough support for day hikes, and can be used in a pinch if your heavier boots prove to be too uncomfortable to wear.

For the more advanced mountaineer, there are double boots. Double boots are the foot's equivalent of a bulldozer and the people wearing them usually mean business. Backpacking guru Colin Fletcher, author of *The Complete Walker,* has coined them "Das Boot." Built with an insulated inner boot and a rigid plastic outer boot, they are the heaviest duty of the boots available. Extreme mountaineers use them for climbing the world's highest and coldest peaks. Their molded plastic shell allows you to attach crampons and front point up ice walls. Double boots are the warmest boots on the market. Of course they are more expensive, heavier, and—never mind what oxygen-deprived high-altitude alpinists tell you—are much less comfortable than leather boots.

*Figure 3-1 Boot Features*

| Boot Model | Features | Use | Price |
|---|---|---|---|
| Double Boot | Molded plastic outer shell, insulated inner boot, aggressive sole, crampon groove | Extreme mountaineering | $200–$500 |
| Rough Trail | Full-grain leather uppers, stiff shank, hefty ankle support, aggressive sole | Long trips with a heavy pack and tough terrain | $175–$300 |
| Off-Trail Boots | Full-grain leather uppers, rugged sole, above-the-ankle support | Two- to five-day trips with moderate weight packs | $125–$200 |
| Light Hikers or Trail Boots | Fabric-leather construction, flexible sole, lightweight | Day trips or trips with a very light pack. They also make good camp shoes | $50–$150 |

## FITTING YOUR BOOTS

In fitting your boots, bring along the type of socks you plan to use in the mountains. At NOLS we have had the most luck with boots worn and fitted with a medium-weight liner sock next to your foot and a thick wool or polyester sock on the outside. The two pairs of socks pad the foot, reduce friction, and wick moisture away from your foot. Therefore, you may have to wear boots in a size or two larger than your street shoes. A good rule of thumb is to put the boots on with no socks, push your toe to where it is touching the front, and still have a finger's width of space between your heel and the back of the boot. Fit any tighter, and your feet will be squeezed and uncomfortable, not to mention cold. Fit any looser, and you will not have the "feel" for the trail that you need to cross boulder fields and slippery terrain. Spend time walking around the store and try different brands. Every brand has its own individual fit and shape because each company uses different foot models around which to design their boot. Some people have "high volume" feet and require a wider, deeper boot. You may find a size ten in one brand fits well in the length but is too tight on your instep. Try on another brand.

Before you go out on your trip, break in your boots with day hikes or even wear them to work. Try to log at least 20 miles on your new boots before you take them out on your extended trip so you can make sure they fit you well.

## CARE OF YOUR BOOTS

Your leather boots will last longer and your feet will stay drier if you "grease" the boots every so often with a leather conditioner. There are four types of sealants available: oil-based, wax-based, silicone-based, and fluoropolymer-based. Recent reviews done by *Backpacker* magazine* suggest that each of these bases can be an effective sealant, but there are big differences in quality between brand names. Nikwax Aqueous Wax, Kiwi Camp Dry, and Tectron Boot/Shoe Protector are reputable and proven products. Be sure to apply the sealant to the tight spots such as where the sole meets the upper.

One of the worst things you can do to a good pair of leather boots is to dry them right by your campfire or next to any powerful heat source. The heat can destroy the boots' glue and degrade the leather. Dry your boots gradually.

# Stoves

For the modern outdoorsperson, lightweight camping stoves are no longer an option, they are a necessity. They make cooking easier and they help protect the local environment. Cooking on a stove is easier than cooking on a fire simply because you can regulate your heat with the turn of a knob, rather than by constantly feeding and monitoring a fire, plus a stove allows you to cook in tight spaces sheltered from the wind, snow, or rain. If everyone were to cook on fires, popular areas would soon be stripped of all their firewood. Some areas already have been plucked clean of the reachable branches and the dead wood on the ground. With a stove, you can cook on a rock or durable surface and leave practically no sign that you were ever there. If that isn't enough to convince you to use a camp stove, consider this: More than a third of national parks require visitors to use stoves rather than campfires.

What qualities do you want in your backpacking stove? Ideally, you want a stove that lights easily, can burn various types of fuel—from white gas to kerosene—boil a quart of water in just a few minutes, simmer on a low heat while you bake, and never fail.

## TYPES OF STOVES

The first decision you have to make when you buy a stove is what sort of fuel it burns. Camping stoves fall into one of two basic categories: multifuel

---

*Backpacker,* August 1997, pp. 66–73.

stoves that burn a variety of liquid fuels such as white gas and kerosene; and stoves that burn only pressurized gas such as isobutane. Multifuel stoves have several advantages over their counterparts that burn pressurized gas. First of all, it's just plain easier to find liquid fuel. Take, for example, the MSR WhisperLite Internationale 600. It burns white gas, kerosene, jet fuel, and auto gasoline. I don't care if you're in Peru or the Punjab, chances are you can find one of those fuels for your camping trip. But try to find a canister of isobutane in one of the more exotic reaches, and you may be out of luck. I once arrived at a particularly remote trailhead only to discover I had forgotten my white gas. The solution was simple—siphon gasoline from my truck and enjoy a slightly more volatile camping trip.

Multifuel stoves are more powerful than isobutane stoves. The benchmark measurement for stove testing is boil time, the time it takes to bring one quart of room temperature water to a boil. Whereas the fastest multifuel stoves have a boil time of about 3.5 minutes, isobutane stoves take up to 30 percent longer to boil that same quart of water. The power differences are magnified in very cold weather, where multifuel stoves perform considerably better than isobutane stoves.

Multifuel stoves are cheaper to run. Per unit dollar, you get between three and four times as much burn time. If you just go camping once or twice a

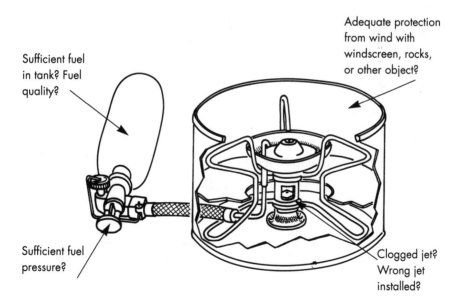

Sufficient fuel in tank? Fuel quality?

Adequate protection from wind with windscreen, rocks, or other object?

Sufficient fuel pressure?

Clogged jet? Wrong jet installed?

Today's multifuel stoves are light, efficient, and easy to use. If your stove isn't running properly, check on these possible problem areas.

year, that's not really an issue, but if you run an outdoor education program or a summer camp, the price difference could add up.

But isobutane stoves do have some advantages. They are simpler to use, generally simmer better for cooking, and are cleaner. You simply attach a fuel canister to the stove, open the valve, and, bingo, you have a nice clean flame. Per unit calorie, isobutane is also lighter than liquid fuels.

## TYPES OF FUELS

### White Gas

The best fuel for your multifuel stove, if you can find it, is always white gas. In the United States and Canada you can easily find white gas in hardware stores, sporting goods stores, and grocery stores under common brands such as Coleman and CampLite. White gas burns cleanly and won't clog or corrode your stove's fuel lines.

### Kerosene

Kerosene is relatively cheap and can be found in much of the world, but it does not burn as cleanly as white gas, leaves more soot, and is more difficult to prime. If you burn kerosene you will have to clean your stove more frequently.

### Automobile Gas

Automobile gas works in a pinch but should only be used when you can't find white gas or kerosene. It is more volatile than either white gas or kerosene and has additives that clog the fuel line and corrode the stove.

*Figure 3-2 Names for Fuel in Other Languages**

| USA | Germany | UK | Australia | France | Italy | Spain | Sweden |
|---|---|---|---|---|---|---|---|
| White gas | Reinbenzin | White gas | Shellite | Essence C | Benzina bianca | Bencina blanca | Ren bensin |
| Kerosene | Petrol | Paraffin | Kerosene | Pétrole | Kerosene | Keroseno | Fotogen |
| Diesel | Diesel | Diesel | Diesel | Gas oil | Gasolio per autotrazióne | Gasóleo automación | Diesel |
| Automobile gas | Autobenzin Z.B. | Petrol | Petrol | Essence normale | Benzina per autoveícoli | Gasolina automación | Bil bensin |

*Source: Mountain Safety Research

## STOVE TROUBLESHOOTING GUIDE*

### Erratic Performance

Insufficient priming

Too much pressure in the fuel bottle

Poor quality or old fuel

Wrong jet installed (MSR specific)

Weather conditions cooling burner. Use windscreen or shelter to protect stove from the wind.

Less oxygen at high altitude. Lower the pressure in the fuel bottle and open the windscreen.

Sooty burner. Wipe soot off flame spreader and burner.

### Reduced Performance

Not enough pressure in the fuel bottle

Clogged jet (usually caused by poor fuel quality)

Wrong jet installed

Fuel is low in bottle

### Pump Not Pressurizing

Dry leather pump cup

Dirt in check valve assembly

▾ Use the best and cleanest fuel available. Fuel loses its potency over a period of just a few months.

▾ Keep your stove clean. Avoid setting it in sand.

# Sleeping Bags

When you decide to buy a sleeping bag, remember that you will spend about a third of your camping trip cocooned inside it. This is, unfortunately, another piece of gear that you can't skimp on. In extreme situations, be it high altitude, unseasonably cold weather, or a case of mild hypothermia, your sleeping bag may save your life. Normally it just means the difference between being comfortable and miserable.

Sleeping bags come in different lengths, weights, and materials. Probably the most important choices to make center around insulation materials.

*Source: Mountain Safety Research

Sleeping bags are insulated with either goose down or one of a variety of types of polyester. Polyester fills include continuous filament fibers like Polarguard 3D; short staple insulations like Primaloft; and the more economical but heavier synthetics like Holofil. The big difference between continuous-filament insulation and short-fiber insulation is this: Short-fiber insulation is more compactable but loses its loft faster; continuous-filament insulation keeps its loft better over the years but is heavier and takes up more room.

The primary advantages of down bags are that they are lighter than polyester fiber bags, last longer (given proper care), and are more compact. The weight difference between artificial fills and down has been narrowed over the last 10 years, but for two bags of the same temperature rating and the same brand, there is still a 10 to 20 percent weight difference between down and synthetic fills. The same five-pound down bag will compress into a smaller unit than its five-pound fiberfill counterpart. Given equal care and equal use, a down bag will keep its insulating properties three or four times as long as polyester bags. A properly cared for down bag might last 20 years, whereas its fiberfill counterpart will usually lose its loft after about five years of regular use. So while down bags are more expensive when you first purchase them, they are less expensive over the long run.

The disadvantage of down is that it takes longer to dry and loses its insulating qualities when wet. When wet, the down feathers clump together, lose their fluff (the term is loft) and their insulating properties as well. Many

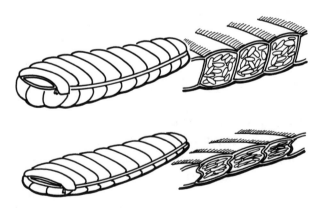

The insulating quality of a sleeping bag depends on trapped air space or "loft." The more loft, the warmer the bag. Down, although an excellent insulator when dry, loses its loft when wet. As a bag ages, it loses its loft and insulating qualities. Storing your bag compressed in a small stuff sack for long periods of time will accelerate the aging of the bag.

down bags now have a Dryloft Gore-Tex shell, which makes them more practical than they were before.

Polyester fiber bags make better bags for wet climates such as the North Cascades and Alaska. The fiber maintains its loft even when wet and, as a result, will still insulate. Polyester fiberfill also dries nearly three times as fast as down.

Bag manufacturers generally use one of four materials for the bag's shell: Dryloft Gore-Tex, microfiber, nylon ripstop, or nylon taffeta. The Dryloft Gore-Tex is the most expensive of the shell materials but has the advantage of being water-resistant (not waterproof) and fairly breathable at the same time. The material is also a good wind breaker. Microfiber also repels water and is breathable. It is not, however, as water-resistant as Dryloft. Nylon ripstop and nylon taffeta are perhaps the two most common sleeping bag shell materials. Both offer a degree of water resistance and windproofing. Nylon taffeta has a nice smooth feel to the skin but isn't as strong as plain old nylon ripstop.

When you purchase your bag, look closely at the design. The cheapest bags are rectangular sacks and have little art behind their shape. The more expensive bags have been designed to prevent loss of heat through radiation. Areas like the zippers where heat can easily escape have insulating baffles sewn on to them to prevent heat loss. At the top of the bag, you'll see a draft collar, which snugs up around your neck to keep heat in when you roll over in your bag. The quality bags have also been sewn with what's known in the trade as shingled construction—a series of sewn compartments—so that the insulation does not migrate to one corner but rather stays in place and insulates the bag evenly.

Camping bags come in two main shapes: the mummy and the narrow mummy. As the name suggests, the bag is shaped to follow the contours of your body and the result is a lighter, warmer bag. A narrow mummy is more tightly conforming than the mummy. The reason not to buy a narrow mummy bag has to do with you and tight spaces. If you are claustrophobic, it makes more sense to buy a standard mummy bag.

Bags also come in different lengths, ranging from about 70 to 90 inches. The best way to find the size and shape for your liking is to try the thing on at the store. Many camping stores will let you actually get the bag out and get inside it. You want your bag to be just big enough to allow about two to five inches of foot room when you are fully inside it. With more room you will not stay as warm at night because you will have to heat up dead air space with your body temperature. Any smaller and you will be uncomfortable. Try on different brands to find a shape that best fits your body shape. You may find the cut of some brands too confining or too generous. Incidentally, some companies now make sleeping bags especially designed for women. They are cut slightly wider in the hip area and slightly narrower in the shoulder area.

Bags also have different insulation ratings. Lightweight bags are rated to between 40 and 50 degrees F, midweight bags are rated to around 20 degrees F, while heavyweight bags can be rated to minus 30 degrees F. Just remember that these ratings should be used just to give you an idea of the bag's weight and loft. The insulation ratings are calculated differently by each company. A North Face bag rated to minus 30 degrees is not necessarily the same as a Marmot bag rated to minus 30 degrees. What's more, you should not assume that because the manufacturer has rated its bag to minus 30 degrees you will necessarily stay warm at that temperature. How warm you are in your bag depends on a number of factors, including your metabolism, what you eat before bed, and the clothing you wear.

Proper care of your sleeping bag will ensure that your investment holds its value. Do not store it for long periods in a compression sack or it will lose its loft. Hang it or store in a cloth bag large enough so that the bag is not compressed. Every time you wash your bag—synthetic or down—it loses some of its life. Obviously you have to wash your bag from time to time, but don't overdo it. Some people sleep in long underwear tops and bottoms to keep the insides of their bags clean. Wash your bag only in a large front-loading washer. The spindle in top-loading washers can damage them.

# Sleeping Pads

Your sleeping bag is only half the equation for a good night's sleep in the backcountry. A good sleeping pad completes the package not only by cush-

*Figure 3-3 Temperature Ratings for Sleeping Bags*

| Temperature Rating | Use |
| --- | --- |
| 30 to 50 degrees F | Warm-weather camping; use in mild climates (e.g., a trip to Lake Powell in early September) |
| 10 to 30 degrees F | Three-season use in moderate climates (e.g., camping in the Sierras, Cascades, or Rockies between May and October) |
| −10 to 10 degrees F | Winter camping, late fall or early spring camping (e.g., a ski trip in Colorado) |
| −50 to −10 degrees F | Extreme mountaineering, polar expeditions (e.g., an ascent of Annapurna) |

ioning you from the sometimes hard, lumpy campsite, but by insulating your body from the cold ground as well. Pads come in two basic varieties: closed-cell foam or self-inflating air-mattresses. You can still buy open-celled foam pads but there's little advantage aside from their low price. As the name suggests, open-celled pads absorb water like a sponge. Closed-cell pads are cheaper than self-inflating pads and can be had for as little as $10. They're also lighter than the air mattresses—usually weighing in at less than a pound. The other good thing about closed-cell foam pads is that there's little to go wrong with them aside from being blown away in a gust of wind. Put more bluntly, they don't leak. Closed-cell pads can also be used in first-aid scenarios for effective splinting and padding.

Self-inflating pads, while more expensive ($50 to $100), heavier (1 to 4 pounds), and prone to puncture, are much more comfortable and warmer. A well inflated air pad really protects you from the bumps in the ground and is a nice, civilized touch for the cold nights. You do have to be more careful with the air pads and avoid the sharp spines and rocks that might puncture them. Be sure to carry a repair kit as well, because if they do get punctured they're not much better than sleeping right on the hard ground. If you pack your self-inflating pad on the outside of your pack, put it in a stuff sack to protect it from the sharp branches along the trail.

Both types of pads come in different sizes, ranging from about 48 inches to about 80 inches. The longer ones obviously cost more and weigh more.

# Packs

The first packs were made of stiff wood frames with little correspondence to the human form. They resembled medieval torture racks and were best suited for those Teutons who took the "no pain, no gain" catchphrase a bit too literally. Had there been no improvement in design over the last thirty years, the backcountry would probably still be empty.

Equipment manufacturers have made great advances in pack design since then. They switched from wood frames to aluminum frames in the sixties, and added a hipbelt to take the weight off the shoulders. In the late 1970s, designers began building packs with flat-metal frames sewn right into the pack bag. The idea was, and still is, that the internal frame could be built to hug the contours of your body and also bring the pack weight in closer to your center of gravity.

Designers modified the frames with lumbar curves, and added sculpted hipbelts, broad shoulder straps, and movable chest straps to better fit the human form. The result? Today packs are much more comfortable and handy than packs of the past.

One thing to remember is that no pack, not even the most gracefully designed one, will be totally comfortable when you are carrying a very heavy load. When I'm going down the trail and the shoulder straps are digging in and the hipbelt won't sit on my hips, I try to think of Nepalese Sherpas carrying their enormous loads with nothing but a tump line. It helps with the pain.

The internal frame pack has supplanted the external frame pack over the last 15 years. For most experienced backpackers, skiers, and mountaineers it is the pack of choice because its design makes carrying a heavy load less awkward than frame packs of the past. With the internal frame pack, the load is moved closer to the body, allowing for more agility, and is more compact.

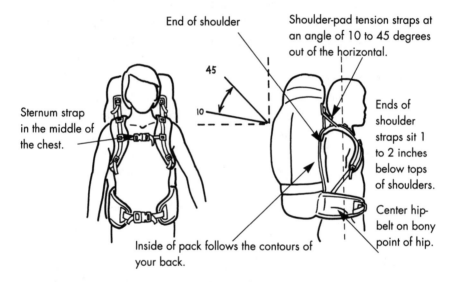

End of shoulder

Shoulder-pad tension straps at an angle of 10 to 45 degrees out of the horizontal.

45

10

Sternum strap in the middle of the chest.

Ends of shoulder straps sit 1 to 2 inches below tops of shoulders.

Center hip-belt on bony point of hip.

Inside of pack follows the contours of your back.

When fitting a pack, load it with about 30 pounds of weight to approximate trail conditions. Every pack is different, but most allow you to adjust the hipbelt and sternum strap vertically, and some allow adjusting of the shoulder yoke vertically as well. Begin by putting the pack on with the hipbelt in its lowest position. Center the hipbelt on the pointed bones of your hips and then adjust the shoulder straps so they are just snug. If your pack has hipbelt trim straps, snug them up. Lightly tighten the shoulder-pad tension straps (also called the lifter straps). Check for the following points of proper fit: The inside of the pack should follow the contours of your back; the upper end of the shoulder pads should sit about one to two inches below the tops of your shoulders; the shoulder stabilizer straps should form an angle of between 10 and 45 degrees from the horizontal. Depending on your pack, you will need to adjust the shoulder yoke, the hipbelt height, and the shoulder stabilizer straps until your pack matches these points of a correct fit. Finally, with the hipbelt and shoulder straps in their correct positions, snug the sternum strap. It should cross the middle of your chest.

But there seems to be a renaissance in frame packs. In a recent conversation I had with Dana Gleason, founder and owner of Dana Packs, he said, "I'm most excited about the future of external frame packs. We have only developed about 30 percent of the potential of external frames whereas we have probably developed about 90 percent of the future of internal frames." Gleason believes the best components of internal frame packs, such as molded hipbelts and compression straps, can and will be incorporated into external frame packs to give hikers a cooler, more comfortable pack. Recent magazine reviews of the newest external frame packs have been favorable.

## CHOOSING A PACK

When choosing your pack, you have to make four basic decisions: external versus internal frame; the volume of the pack; the size of the pack frame; and the brand.

### External Frames versus Internal Frames

The table below summarizes the advantages and disadvantages of external frame packs and internal frame packs. Most instructors I know at NOLS

*Figure 3-4 External vs. Internal Frame Packs*

|  | Pros | Cons |
| --- | --- | --- |
| External Frame Pack | ▾ High center of gravity makes it easier to walk upright<br>▾ Air flow between pack and body makes for cooler hiking<br>▾ Easier to load<br>▾ Cheaper than internal frame packs<br>▾ Won't sag under heavy loads<br>▾ Frame can be used to make a litter to evacuate injured party | ▾ High center of gravity makes it harder to balance in tricky terrain or when skiing<br>▾ Doesn't move as closely to your body, making it harder to scramble over obstacles<br>▾ More bulky for air travel |
| Internal Frame Pack | ▾ Pack rides low and close to the body, allowing you freedom of movement and better balance<br>▾ Sleek profile makes it easier to bushwhack, crawl through tight boulder fields, etc. | ▾ More difficult to load and pack<br>▾ More expensive than external frame packs<br>▾ Not useful for making litters |

use an internal frame pack because of the terrain they have to cross leading courses. The internal frame pack fits closer to the body and allows better balance. Most pack manufacturers have put their effort into developing the internal frame pack over the last ten years and it shows in the design improvements that it has undergone.

The table below summarizes pack volumes and corresponding uses.

*Figure 3-5 Pack Volume According to Use*

| Intended Use | Pack Size (in cubic inches) |
| --- | --- |
| Day hiking | 3,000 |
| Single-day rock climbing/single-day backcountry skiing | 4,000 |
| Backpacking trips of five days or less | 5,000 |
| Backpacking of more than five days | 6,000–7,000 |
| Long expeditions with extensive gear/Backpacking trips of more than a week | 6,000+ |

## PACK PACKING

Some hikers string water bottles, cups, shoes, and sundry other items from their packs with string or cord and walk down the trail looking like the getaway car for newlyweds. Their gear makes a noisy clanking and a water bottle or something seems to fly the coop at every turn in the trail. Aside from making the pack ungainly, snagging on bushes, making a racket, and slowing the group with reassembly, packing this way plain looks bad. Naturally there will be times when you can't fit everything into your pack and you need to lash something onto the outside. But think it through a bit, pick an item like a foam pad or a fishing rod—something that won't snag on trees and that can be tightly lashed to your pack. And then lash it on tightly. Every trip is different and every pack will be different. But if you follow certain principles in pack packing, you will build something infinitely more beautiful and balanced. Some NOLS instructors use the mnemonic ABC to teach pack packing. A stands for accessibility, B for balance, and C for compactness.

**Accessibility.** As a backpacker, you need to keep certain things accessible. In some cases it's just a matter of convenience and consideration for your campmates. No one likes to wait five minutes every time the budding pho-

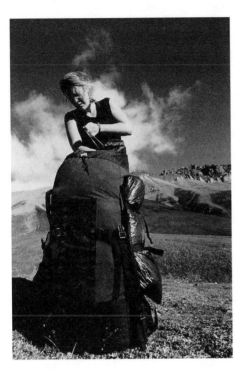

NOLS instructor Eleanor Huffines packing her pack on a NOLS trip in Alaska's Brooks Range. A well-packed pack is balanced and compact. Try to get everything to fit inside the pack by filling the small spaces (such as empty pots and mugs) with odd items such as clothing and food. *Tom Bol*

tographer in the group dismantles his entire pack to fish out the Nikon. Start with clothing. In the mountains or the desert the weather can change in a hurry. We all know the old refrain, "If you don't like the weather, wait a minute." Keep an extra warm layer, a wind layer, and a waterproof layer handy. Here are some other things you may want to keep accessible: sunscreen, water bottle, snack food, first aid supplies, camera, sunglasses, sun hat.

**Balance.** A well-packed, balanced pack of 50 pounds will be easier to carry than an unbalanced pack of 40 pounds. If your pack is top-heavy, it will be hard to keep your balance crossing logs or negotiating boulder fields. A pack with too much weight at the bottom will hinder your stride. The key is to pack the dense heavy things in close to your body and at a level between your shoulder blades and the bottom of your rib cage. Things like food, the tent, and the radio (if you carry one) are good items to carry in the mid-regions of your pack.

**Compactness.** If you have a huge pack and are going out for only a few days, you will have plenty of room to fit all your gear. But if you plan to camp for more than about five days, you have to pack well to utilize limited space.

## Things You'll Be Tempted to Bring but Can Do Without

▾ Deodorant: No one smells like a rose out in the wilds, nor should you.

▾ Shampoo and conditioner: These are just extra weight. If you want to wash your hair use a little soap.

▾ A 12-inch combat sheath knife: Unless you plan on skinning a large ungulate, these are heavy and a waste of space. A small pocket knife is all you need around the kitchen.

▾ Too many changes of clothes: You can get by without that second or third T-shirt and a change of underwear for every day of your trip.

▾ Oversized toiletries: Instead of bringing a huge tube of toothpaste, squeeze a little into an old plastic film canister. Instead of a huge hairbrush, maybe just a small plastic comb will do.

What's more, the compact pack will be less ungainly to carry. You can take better advantage of space in your pack by breaking large units down into smaller units. Your tent will pack more densely if you pack the fly separately from the tent body. Food, too, can be crammed into the small empty spaces rather than trying to put all your food in one large bag. Look for items like pots, pans, and cups that have lots of dead space and fill them up with clothing or food. Some items such as sleeping bags and clothing can be compressed to half their volume with compression sacks. Once everything is all packed, take advantage of your pack's compression straps (if your model has them) and cinch the pack down tightly.

### Other Packing Tips

▾ Waterproof your sleeping bag and clothes by lining a nylon stuff sack with a heavy-duty garbage bag. Waterproof small items such as your extra maps with zip-lock bags.

▾ Use nylon bags with zippers and small stuff sacks to organize your pack and ultimately your life while out in the mountains. You'll develop your own organization scheme, but here are a few examples of things to keep in one stuff sack: warm clothing for the camp such as dry socks, long underwear, hat, and gloves; assorted items that you only need around camp such as eating utensils, extra flashlight batteries, a book, and toiletries; repair items such as a stove repair kit, extra nylon cord, and ripstop nylon.

▾ Always pack your food above your fuel. Good fuel bottles rarely leak, but if they ever do, you don't want the fuel giving your granola an octane rating.

Pack heavy, dense items like food close into the body and over the middle part of your back (between the rib cage and the shoulder blades). Shorter people may feel more comfortable with the food lower in the pack (just above sleeping bag).

Odd items such as camp shoes can be used to fill up small spaces.

Water kept in easily accessible place to help keep yourself hydrated.

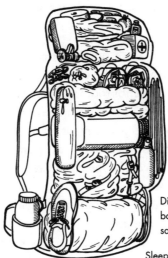

Items like maps, first aid supplies, lunch, a warm layer of clothing, and a headlamp should be kept accessible in the top or outside pockets.

Fill hollow spaces like the insides of pots and pans with small odd items to save on space.

Pack fuel below the food in case of a spill.

Dismantle and pack tent fly, body, and poles separately to save on space.

Sleeping bag on the bottom. Line stuff sack with large garbage bag to waterproof pack.

Think of the ABCs when packing: accessibility, balance, and compactness.

# Tents

On the best trips, trips when the weather treats you kindly, you don't have to spend much time in your tent. But if the weather goes foul, a good tent is your best friend. Mountaineering lore is rich with stories of being tent bound at the base of some horrendous route for days as a storm hammers its way through. Rick Ridgeway, author of *The Shadow of Kilimanjaro,* and a member of the first successful American ascent of K2, reckons he has spent literally three or four years of his life in a tent. I would estimate that senior NOLS instructors have spent even more time there. There's no cozier place than the confines of a good tent in a big storm, and there's no place more miserable than in a leaky tent at midnight when the heavens let loose.

There are some excellent tents on the market. The best tents have been tested in the factory but more importantly in the field by outdoor professionals. The best companies test their tents in the world's worst conditions: Mount Washington, for instance. Tent manufacturers go so far as to build rain rooms, where the tent is hammered by 500 gallons of water per minute for days on end. The best tents are easy to set up, can take an eighty-mile-an-hour wind, hold steady under a foot of snow, and don't weigh very much, all things considered.

## TYPES OF TENTS

### Shapes

The first camping tents were simple A-frames. They had rigid poles at each end, and were a version of one of the oldest shelter designs in history. The A-frame offered little interior room relative to the amount of fabric used, and except for the lucky person sleeping in the center, they offered little head room. What's more, their steep, unsupported walls met the wind square on and could be flattened by strong gusts. The A-frame tent should not be your choice of tent unless you want to reenact a Civil War battle or host a slumber party in your living room.

There are two basic tent designs on the market today: the dome tent and the hoop or tunnel tent. The dome tent is the strongest and most versatile tent and is the best choice for the average outdoorsperson. As the name suggests, it is dome shaped and was modeled after the late Buckminster Fuller's geodesic dome. Through a combination of flexed aluminum poles, a reinforced nylon body, and very clever architecture, designers have come up with a lightweight structure that can take a whipping in the wind, rain, and snow. Dome tents have a high volume to fabric ratio, which means you have more head room. The best dome tents have a streamlined design that sheds the wind. Dome tents are self-standing, which means you can assemble the body, pick it up, and move it to the best site, then attach the fly and stake the whole thing down.

Hoop tents have some of the same design features of dome tents but use fewer poles and less fabric per unit-person. As a result, they are lighter but not quite as strong. You might choose a hoop tent for summer camping or areas of the world where high winds and/or heavy snows are unlikely. If you have to shave pounds—traveling solo or bicycling, perhaps—the hoop tent may be a good selection as well.

### Single-Wall versus Double-Wall Tents

Most tents on the market come in two parts: the canopy and the fly. The canopy, except for the polyurethane-coated floor, is made with uncoated nylon to allow moisture passage. The fly is made of a polyurethane-coated nylon and is intended to be waterproof. The theory is that the breathable walls allow the moisture from your respiration, sweat, or wet gear to pass through the canopy out to the fly, where it condenses and slides harmlessly down the inside of the fly to the ground. The fly provides the waterproof barrier from rain and snow. The double-wall design works well though not perfectly. In the extreme cold, the moisture from inside your tent can freeze on the canopy and create a layer of frost. If the tent is poorly made, or poorly pitched, for that matter, the fly can sag onto the canopy and the condensation will likely drip on your party all night.

To increase ventilation and keep your canopy drier, some double-wall tent designs include what are called "low-high" vents. The idea is that warm moist air flows out the high vents and is replaced by cool dry air entering the low vents. The vents do help air circulation and keep you drier provided the weather isn't too harsh. But if you're camping in snow, moisture can enter the low vents.

Single-wall tents, by contrast, are usually made of three-layer nylon laminates that allow moisture to escape from within but keep water from entering from without. The idea behind single-wall tents is that they are easier to pitch and lighter. Naturally they are more expensive than their double-wall counterpart. The trouble with single-wall tents is that they tend to condense inside and have a muggy feel to them in hot weather. They also require more maintenance: You have to keep their seams well seam-sealed or they leak.

### For Every Season a Tent

Tents can be further divided into three-season tents and four-season tents. Three-season tents, as the name suggests, will get you through the spring, summer, and fall. But if you want to winter camp or climb extreme mountains, you will need a four-season tent. Four-season tents are about 10 to 15 percent heavier than three-season tents, have a more rigid frame structure, a large vestibule (for cooking or gear storage), and are made with heavier fabric.

## TENT SIZES

Tent sizes vary from company to company. A typical two-person tent will have a floor area between 30 and 40 square feet; a three-person tent will typically have a floor area between 40 and 50 square feet; and a four-person tent will have a floor with an area of between 50 and 60 square feet. If possible, set the tent up in the store to get a feel for the size (and the complexity of assembly). In general, a three-person tent will hold three people—but snugly. If you can carry the extra weight, bring a tent with the capacity to hold one more person than the total number in your group, and you'll have extra room for gear and your sleeping bag.

The other factor to consider is the size of the tent's vestibule. The ves-

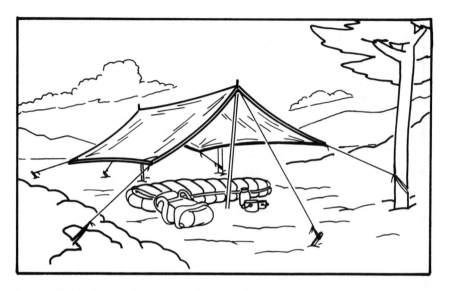

A simple fly like the one shown in this illustration has certain advantages over a tent: It's lighter, less expensive, and can be pitched over irregular surfaces that might cut the floor of a tent.

tibule is an extension of the tent's roof and is designed to protect gear from the weather and give campers a place to shed wet gear. Some tents have a vestibule of 20 square feet while other tents have no vestibule at all. The vestibule is a nice touch—sort of like a mud room—and frees up some space in the tent's interior.

### FLIES

Many NOLS courses forgo tents for just a fly. These are not simply the fly from a double-wall tent, but a specially cut tarp. Flies have several advantages over tents and certainly some shortcomings as well. With just two poles and a roof, they are considerably lighter and cheaper. You can set them up in areas where you can't set up a tent because you don't have to worry about sharp objects cutting the floor. Flies also have a nice airy, outdoorsy feeling and can be pitched to make a nice shady area on hot days. If you use a fly, you should bring a ground cloth to sleep on.

Flies are not as good as tents for very cold, very wet, or very windy weather. Because a tent fully encloses the campers and creates a dead air space, it is much warmer than a fly. Even the very best pitched fly will not shelter you from the rain, snow, and wind like a high-quality tent. The other thing about flies: They don't keep the mosquitoes out.

## Tips on Pitching Your Tent

▾ Don't overestimate your weather prediction skills. The most peaceful afternoons can deteriorate quickly into wet storms. Pitch your tent with pessimism.

▾ Study the site. Avoid subtle depressions that will become lakes if it rains. Watch for sharp sticks and rocks that can put a hole in your tent's floor.

▾ Find a sheltered area. You'll stay much warmer sheltered from the wind, and your tent has a better chance of making it through the night.

▾ Use as many tie-out points as possible to give your tent strength.

▾ Use buried sticks for anchor points when camped in snow. Loop the cord around the stick and bury it in the snow (harden the snow by stomping on it a few times) and then tie the cord off at the tent.

▾ If you use rocks for anchor points, use big ones—at least the size of a basketball—so they bear up against a strong wind.

## PITCHING YOUR TENT

The strength of your tent does of course depend on the construction, design, and quality, but it also depends on how well you pitch it. If you erect even the sturdiest of tents on an unprotected ridge and don't do a good job staking it out, a high wind can shred it. Try to find the most sheltered area, whether in a group of trees, behind a rock, or behind a snow wall you yourself construct. Once pitched, make the tent taut with the various tie-downs provided by the designer. Not only will a taut tent be stronger, it will better shed rain and snow.

Putting a ground cloth below your tent's floor will make your tent last longer, although carrying a ground cloth adds weight to your pack. If you don't have a ground cloth, avoid sharp rocks and sticks that might tear the floor.

## CARE AND MAINTENANCE OF YOUR TENT

Ultraviolet light and water are arguably the two greatest dangers to the life of your tent. That may sound absurd given the fact that your tent lives in the sun and the rain when you go out camping. But the real danger from the sun and water come not so much when you go out for a weekend or even a week, but from improper storage. The best thing to do when you come home from a camping trip is to wash your tent with a sponge and water. Then dry it thoroughly. If you store your tent wet, the combination of room-temperature heat, dirt, and water can lead to bacterial growth and the breakdown of the tent's outer coating. Store your tent loosely in an oversized, breathable bag so if any condensation forms from a temperature change, the moisture can easily evaporate.

Your tent's poles are ideally stored fully assembled. Extended, the shock

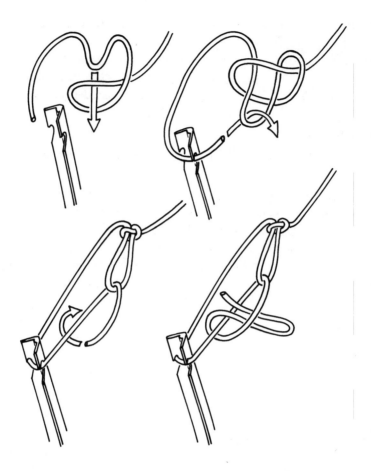

The trucker's hitch is a great thing to have in your quiver of tricks. It's often the first knot we teach students on NOLS courses to use for pitching a tent. It is simple to tie, easy to adjust, and easy to untie. Because it forms a pulley and gives you a 3 to 1 mechanical advantage, it can be used to cinch items down on your pack, to raise heavy food bags for bear hangs, or just to tie your gear to the roof rack of your car on your way to the mountains.

cord in the poles takes less stress. You may not have the room to store them extended, but even storing them loosely in a large bag will make the shock cord last longer. When disassembling your tent, break the poles apart from the middle and work your way outward rather than starting at one end; it places less stress on the shock cords.

Before you go on your trip, be sure to seam-seal the tent. Seam-seal is a silicon compound that waterproofs the seams, which are vulnerable to leakage due to the stitching. The new seam-seals can be applied to the outside of the tent.

The most vulnerable part of a tent is the zipper. Pull too hard on your zipper and suddenly you don't have the option of shutting the door should it ever snow or get really cold. If your zipper jams, be gentle with it.

### Tips on Zippers

- ▾ Putting a little candle wax or even lip balm helps lubricate your zipper. You can also buy commercial lubricant for zippers.
- ▾ If your zipper does not close, check to make sure there is not undue tension on it from the fabric. Try to relieve some of the tension by pulling the sides closer together before zipping it.
- ▾ Use two hands to open and close zippers.
- ▾ Clean with a toothbrush or nail brush if the zipper gets mud or grit in it.
- ▾ Bring along spare zipper pulls and know how to replace them.

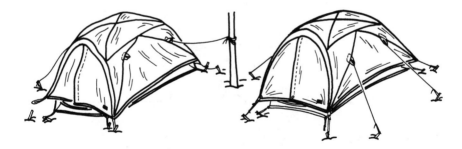

The well-pitched tent (right) will likely keep you drier in a storm and last longer as well. When tightly pitched, a tent is stronger and more aerodynamic than a loose and sagging tent. Use all your tie-outs and stakeout points. Wet cord stretches, so be vigilant about retightening the tie-outs. Pity the inhabitants of the tent on the left should a powerful storm develop.

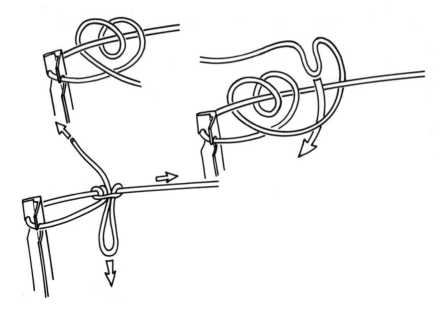

The slippery taut line is an effective knot for staking out your tent. It is simple to tie and allows you to adjust the tension on the lines.

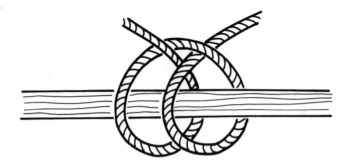

The clove hitch is one of the most useful hitches for outdoor travelers. It's an adjustable hitch that can be used to secure a lash strap on a frame pack, keep a tent or fly line from slipping down a supporting pole, tie a boat to a pole, or jerry-rig a pack saddle. Experiment with this hitch and you'll find it has a lot of uses.

### Interview with John Roskelley

John Roskelley, widely considered to be one of the world's premier mountaineers, was on the first American teams to summit K2 (28,250 feet), Makalu (27,800 feet), Dhaulagiri (26,780 feet), and Nanda Devi (25,640 feet), all without bottled oxygen. Roskelley has pioneered some of the most challenging alpine routes including Gaurishankar. He is the author of *Stories off the Wall*, *Last Days*, and *Nanda Devi: The Tragic Expedition*. Roskelley lives in Spokane, Washington.

**Q:** What has most helped you achieve your goals?

**A:** My partners. Mountaineering is not an individual sport. Your partners are the number one criteria for success. It comes down to who you're with. Your partners bolster your courage and support you when you need it.

**Q:** What do you look for in choosing a teammate or partner?

**A:** Experience; safety record; consistency in success, which indicates all of the above. One rule of thumb: If their shoes don't stay tied, I don't go with them.

**Q:** What is the most overrated advice about mountaineering or traveling in the backcountry?

**A:** That you need all the gear they try to sell you at the sporting-goods stores. Anything fancier than normal is marketing. A lot of mountains were climbed with simple stuff throughout the years. I just took a group of trekkers/climbers to Ladakh in northern India. One of them came with every conceivable piece of equipment and it didn't help. Keep it to the basics.

**Q:** What to you is the most important piece of equipment not including technical gear?

**A:** Your pack, headlamp, and proper-fitting footgear. These are simple things, but more people screw up on the simple things than on major items. People spend all the time in the world making sure their crampons are adjusted just right and then they forget something as simple as their headlamp.

**Q:** What advances in equipment over the last 15 years help you most?

**A:** Polar pile gear. It's lightweight, dries quickly, and is durable. Wool still keeps you dry when wet, but it's like wearing a suit of chain mail. And down. You might as well be wearing a wind jacket if it gets soaked. There certainly won't be any insulation value.

**Q:** What is an example of simple gear you use instead of the fancy stuff?

**A:** Running shoes. I hike in trail running shoes right up to the point on the glacier where I have to put on my crampons.

**Q:** What advice would you give someone about traveling efficiently and safely in the backcountry?

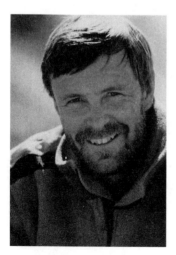

John Roskelley, considered by many to be the most successful American mountaineer.

**A:** Know your limitations and listen to your inner self. Use some judgment. If it doesn't feel right, then you probably shouldn't be there. If it doesn't feel right then back off.

**Q:** What appeals to you about the backcountry?

**A:** The wildlife and getting away from too many people.

# Water Systems

Some pack companies make inexpensive "dromedary" systems that allow you to have a drink of water without unloading your whole pack. The system costs about $20 and is simply a Mylar bag inside a nylon pouch, and a plastic tube to drink from. You fill the bag with water, put it in the top pocket of your pack, and then drink from the tube at your convenience. I use this sort of system for bicycling, cross-country skiing, and backpacking. Because it's so easy to get a drink—no fussing with my pack—I drink more water and stay better hydrated. You can also just bring a plastic water bottle if you like. Bring at least one one-quart bottle, and two if you are traveling in the desert or in an area where water sources are scarce.

A collapsible water jug or water bag with a two- to three-gallon capacity is a big help in the kitchen. They don't weigh much but can save you lots of time and trouble. At times when you have to camp a great distance from water, these jugs will save you from having to shuttle pots of water back and forth from the river or lake. There are a few different models on the market, ranging from the inexpensive plastic accordion-style to the more expensive urethane-coated nylon bags, the latter of which can be set up for a makeshift solar shower.

# Headlamps and Flashlights

To be honest here, I use a headlamp primarily to read trashy mysteries late into the night. But a good headlamp or flashlight is an important piece of equipment that serves in emergencies as well as in common chores in the dark. You can bring just a flashlight, but it's well worth it to spring a few extra bucks for a headlamp. Say you've just had a tough day out on the trail and don't get camp set up until dark. With a headlamp, your hands are free to light the stove, do the cooking, and organize camp. With just a flashlight, you have one hand tied up. Given a complex task, you'll put the flashlight in your mouth, grip it in your teeth, and congratulate yourself on the $10 you saved not buying a headlamp. Buy the best headlamp you can afford and bring extra batteries and an extra bulb. It's worth it. Reverse or remove the batteries in your headlamp when you pack it away for the day so it doesn't inadvertently switch on and use up the batteries.

## Knife or Multipurpose Tool

A small pocketknife or a multipurpose tool like a Leatherman is essential for repairing equipment, cutting parachute cord, and chopping cheese. The key here is to find a knife or tool small enough with just the blades you need. The Swiss Army company makes nice knives with a good assortment of blades. The following blades are the most important ones to have on your knife:

- ▼ Knife blade: for preparing food, cutting leather and nylon, and making wood shavings for a fire.
- ▼ Scissors: for cutting tape and moleskin.
- ▼ Flat-blade screwdriver and Phillips head screwdriver; some piece of equipment will have a loose screw.

The multipurpose tools weigh a bit more than the simple knives but have the distinct advantage of having needlenose pliers incorporated right into the body. Needlenose pliers are so handy that I've taken to carrying a multipurpose tool instead of a knife, as have many NOLS instructors. The pliers come in handy for undoing tough knots, picking up a hot pan, fixing a stove, and bending whatever metal needs bending.

## Equipment Repair

The lucky ones make it through their whole trip with all their gear intact and never have to repair any of it. But sooner or later a piece of gear fails or an article of clothing tears. You would do well to bring along a small repair kit to deal with eventualities. Here is a list of what to take in a small repair kit:

- ▼ Duct tape is good for fixing nearly anything from broken sunglasses to a torn map. You can either bring a small roll or take a length off a big roll

## The Essential Extras

Most seasoned campers have a favorite item they bring outside the list of essentials. Here are a few examples of items you won't find on a typical equipment list that some NOLS instructors nevertheless bring. Don't bring all these; pick and choose carefully.

▾ Wool bandanna (to keep your neck warm)
▾ Sponge to mop out the tent
▾ Leatherman (to fix a stove, use as pot grips, fix a pack, etc.)
▾ Adjustable ski poles for walking sticks
▾ Dental floss and sewing needle (dental floss doubles as thread)
▾ Crazy Creek chair (to sit and reflect; use as a splint; extra padding at night)

and wrap it around your water bottle or—if you bring one—your ski pole.

▾ A speedy stitcher is a most handy tool for repairing packs, boots, and gaiters. The heavy-duty thread and the pattern of stitches makes for very strong repairs.
▾ Ripstop nylon weighs next to nothing and can be used to repair tents, jackets, and wind pants.
▾ A small roll of mechanical wire can be handy to repair packs, certain stoves, and sometimes boots.
▾ Bring a standard sewing kit with strong thread to fix torn clothing.
▾ 20 feet of nylon parachute cord
▾ Extra toggles

# Care of Equipment

Once you have made the investment in good equipment, be, as Wendell Berry puts it, "a true materialist" and take care of your gear. Not only will it last longer, but it will serve you better. What's more, you won't have to replace it as often and you will conserve natural resources. Here are five commandments for equipment care:

I.  Thou shalt not store equipment wet. It will mildew and compromise the materials.
II.  Thou shalt not leave equipment made of synthetic materials in the sun any longer than necessary. The sun is the enemy of most artificial fibers.
III.  Thou shalt keep leather boots well oiled.
IV.  Thou shalt studiously review and update any technical equipment such as ropes, carabiners, and rock protection before hanging thy life on it.
V.  Thou shalt go easy on all zippers, realizing they are delicate, and not force them open or closed without first trying to finesse them.

# Equipment Summary

▾ Look for good, not fancy, equipment. Be skeptical about gadgets.

▾ Your boots, tent, pack, sleeping bag, and stove are the tools that will help you travel safely and comfortably. Whether you buy these items used or new, make sure they are of high quality, good design, and in good condition.

▾ Work toward bringing just the right amount of gear. Too much stuff and you'll bend under the load. Too little of the essential gear and you may have some hard cold nights.

# CHAPTER 4

# How to Dress for the Backcountry

During the Great War, a Turkish army was sent to fight Russia in the snowbound passes of Central Asia. Of the 150,000 Turks, 50,000 froze to death, because, to quote Marshall, they were not "dressed for it."

—Mark Helprin, *The Wall Street Journal*, February 22, 1996

The human condition is not a particularly happy one when it comes to staying warm and dry in the outdoors. While the rest of the world's warm-blooded creatures kept their fur and feathers for a cold rainy day, over a course of some millions of years, we humans shed the bulk of our hair to become, in the words of Desmond Morris, "naked apes." As warm-blooded animals, we need to keep our core temperature up to nearly 100 degrees Fahrenheit. The universe, with its second law of thermodynamics, conspires to bring our core temperature down to its level. Ultimately it's a losing battle, and someday the universe will win. But while we're alive and kicking, we can put on the good fight by dressing appropriately.

When you travel in remote areas, you can't afford to bring a lot of clothes. Your pack can only hold so much and your back has limits too. So you have to choose your clothing wisely. You have to bring as little as possible and still have protection from a storm or a cold day.

On camping trips, the temperature and the weather conditions can change fast. It can snow in June or, conversely, the air temperature on glaciers can heat up to 80 degrees. To complicate matters, your own body heats up and cools off—sometimes radically—depending on what you eat, whether or not you're exerting yourself, your level of hydration, your physical state, and other factors.

Fortunately, with the advances in clothing fabrics in recent decades, keeping warm and dry in the backcountry is a relatively simple proposition. With our clothing we create a microuniverse around our bodies and, done right, become warm, dry islands unto ourselves. The very word insulation comes from the Latin word for island. In this chapter we'll discuss heat loss, clothing materials, layering, and specific clothing items.

## A Short Course in Thermodynamics and Heat Transfer

The second law of thermodynamics states that any object placed in an infinite environment will eventually reach the same temperature as that environment. Simply stated, on a cold day the universe will do its damnedest to chill us to its temperature if we don't dress to prevent it. The universe has a bag of tricks to induce heat loss, including conduction, convection, and radiation. When a cold object is touching a warm object, the cold object becomes warmer and the warm object becomes colder through conduction. In the practical world, when you sit on a cold rock, you lose heat through conduction. Your seat gets colder, the rock you're sitting on gets warmer, and the god of thermodynamics stays happy. If it's a big cold rock, you will eventually be chilled to the temperature of the rock (or a minuscule amount higher) simply because it is a much bigger heat sink than you are.

Certain materials conduct heat better than others. Have you ever drunk coffee out of a metal cup and burned your lips on the rim? That same coffee barely heats up a plastic mug. Metal is a better conductor than plastic; plastic is a better insulator.

When a cold liquid or gas comes into contact with a warm body, the liquid or gas will gain heat and the solid will lose heat. This is convection. If you stand in a cold river the water will chill you through convection; if you sit in a north wind, the air will chill you through convection as well.

The heat you feel when you stand next to a fire travels from the fire to your hands through radiation. Radiation is the transfer of heat through electromagnetic waves. Our bodies radiate heat 24 hours per day.

The backcountry traveler is constantly losing or gaining heat through conduction, convection, and radiation. The skier who grips his cold ski pole without putting on his gloves promptly experiences conduction. The kayaker drenched in a cold river gives up heat through convection. Over the decades of outdoor travel and adventure, clever humans devised numerous ingenious items of apparel to help our furless species resist these universal forces.

# Backcountry Clothing Fabrics

In the good old days, mountaineers dressed in wool socks, wool sweaters, and leather knickers. The truth is, those same clothes still work, and both wool and leather are decent materials for certain purposes. But outdoor clothing companies have developed such excellent synthetic materials that even the diehard naturalists wear a little of the artificial stuff. Now we have polyester in all its incarnations—fleece, pile, and polarguard—various weights and forms of nylon, and high-tech breathable materials such as Gore-Tex. You can wear a broad combination of natural and artificial fibers as long as you keep in mind certain principles.

- ▾ **Cotton** has been used for thousands of years, and today it is still the most common clothing textile. Cotton is a great fabric for hot days when you're primarily concerned with cooling down, not staying warm. It absorbs several times its weight in water and ventilates well. But cotton is a poor choice of fabric for the cold or wet days. Once wet, it not only loses its insulating qualities but also retains water, which is highly conductive. A wet cotton shirt, then, promotes heat loss on a cold day. Cotton also takes a long time to dry.
- ▾ **Wool,** like cotton, absorbs water easily and takes a long time to dry. The difference is that wool maintains tiny air pockets in its interstices even when wet and therefore maintains its insulating values. If you don't mind its itchy qualities, wool can be worn against the skin as a base layer, or you can wear it as an insulating mid-layer.
- ▾ **Down** per unit weight is one of the best insulators available. It also compresses easily so you can pack down clothing into tight spaces. The problem with down is that it collapses when wet and loses the air pockets that make it a good insulator. When wet, down is practically useless as an insulator. If weight and space are of top priority, and you are confident you can keep your clothing dry, nothing beats down for a mid-layer.
- ▾ **Polyester** Clever chemical engineers have in some ways improved on the woolen sheep and the feathered goose with the material we all know as polyester. If you spend much time in the outdoors you'll probably be wearing a lot of the stuff. Polyester is the base for dozens of clothing materials and insulations such as pile, fleece, Lycra, Capilene, and polarguard. Polyester doesn't absorb water and dries quickly. As a result it makes an ideal insulator and/or base layer. For the equivalent warmth, polyester insulation is much lighter than wool.

- ▾ **Nylon** is a strong, abrasion-resistant fabric used for shells, jackets, wind pants, and rain clothes. In its original form it is a breathable material that works well to protect against the wind but not the rain. Coated with polyurethane, nylon can be made into a waterproof fabric.
- ▾ **Gore-Tex** is an ultrathin film that clothing manufacturers laminate onto materials such as nylon. It has literally billions of microscopic pores (9 billion per square inch), large enough to allow passage of water vapor (i.e., vapor from sweat) but not large enough to allow passage of water in its liquid form (i.e., rain and melting snow). The theory is that Gore-Tex allows vapor rising off your body to escape without allowing you to get wet from the rain. Gore-Tex works well to keep the rain and snow out and does allow some vapor to escape. The first problem with Gore-Tex is that it's still very expensive. Expect to pay 50 to 100 percent more for a Gore-Tex item than you would for its nylon counterpart. The second problem with Gore-Tex is that if you're really working hard—climbing a steep trail, for instance—the material doesn't vent fast enough to keep you dry from the inside. You can certainly help the process by opening the vents on your clothing, but the system still hasn't been perfected.

## KNOW THE CLIMATE

To choose the right clothing, whether for your two-day backpack trip or your ascent of Annapurna, you must first understand the climate where you will be traveling. That might sound like obvious advice: If it's cold bring warm clothes and if it's hot bring sunscreen. But every climate has its quirks, and the more you understand those quirks, the more likely it is that you will bring the right gear. Consider the Cascade Mountains and the Rocky Mountains, for instance. Both have rugged alpine terrain rising over ten thousand feet. But the storms in the Cascades—weather straight off the Pacific Ocean—are wet and will soak you. The Rockies are generally drier. So if you travel in western Washington you might want to make sure that all your insulating layers are either synthetic material or wool. In Colorado, you can do okay with insulating layers made from down.

People climbing Mount McKinley usually bring warm sleeping bags and hefty parkas but many forget that the glaciers can be scorching hot in the middle of the day and don't bring the right clothing to travel in the heat. People think of the desert as warm and sandy, but desert nights can freeze the water in your water bottle, and even in late spring the desert has an annoying habit of snowing on your party.

The point is, you should study the area you're visiting and talk to people with first-hand experience so you come prepared for the subtle differences in climes.

# Layering

Consider a typical day on the trail. Early in the morning it's 40 degrees and you're just starting out on a gradual descent. After two miles, the trail begins a steep climb and the sun has brought the temperature up 10 degrees. You climb 3,000 feet to the top of a pass and stop to eat lunch and take in the view. A wind picks up and it begins to drizzle. You scamper down the pass into a forest where by now it is pouring rain.

In that short span of a few hours, think of what has happened to your body temperature as you descended the trail, then climbed a steep pass, then sat and ate lunch, and then descended again. Chances are, your body started cold in the morning, warmed up considerably as you climbed the pass, cooled again when you stopped to rest, warmed a bit with the food you ate

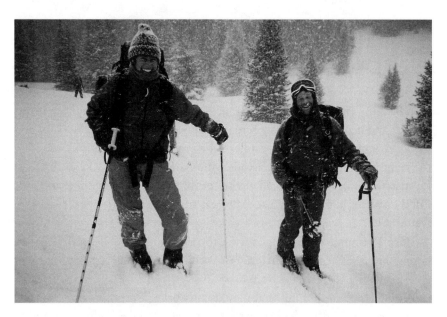

NOLS instructors Abby Warner and Gary Wilmot enjoying a day of backcountry skiing in the Wyoming Range mountains. By dressing with the right clothing layers, they can regulate their body temperatures and stay comfortable despite the snowfall, a cool ambient temperature, and rigorous exercise. *John McConnell*

at lunch, and then cooled as you descended the pass in the rain. To confound all that, the weather changed with the time of day, the altitude, the wind, and the rain. The simplest way to dress for the many changes in body temperature and ambient temperature that one experiences in a typical day on the trail is through layering.

The principles of layering are simple: Layering allows you to microadjust the immediate climate next to your body. A giant down parka and a wool shirt may keep you just as warm as, say, the combination of a lightweight polyester shirt, a midweight shirt, a pile jacket, and a nylon windbreaker, but the former doesn't allow the flexibility of the latter in regulating your temperature. It's akin to having a thermostat in your house with just two settings—off and broiling—versus having the full spectrum of adjustment.

For our purposes, we can divide clothing layers into three groups:

- ▾ Base layer: the layer that actually touches your skin.
- ▾ Intermediate layers: the layers that you put on over the base layer to insulate.
- ▾ Outer layer: the last layer you put on to protect against snow, rain, or wind.

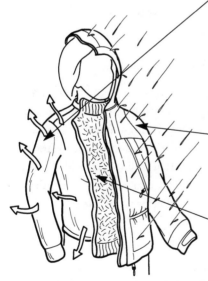

Because the base layer comes in direct contact with your skin, it needs to be made of a material that keeps you warm even when wet. Polyester-based materials like Thermax, CoolMax, and Capilene insulate when wet and also "wick" moisture away from your skin. Wool can be used as a base layer but takes longer to dry and is less comfortable.

The outer layer protects you from the wind and/or rain. It can be a waterproof material like coated nylon, a breathable material like Gore-Tex, or, in the case of windshells, uncoated nylon.

The midlayer insulates. It can be made of wool, a polyester form such as pile or fleece, or down. On very cold days, you may need two or three midlayers.

Dressing in layers of suitable clothing allows you to microadjust the environment around your body and stay comfortable and dry despite what Mother Nature throws in your direction.

## BASE LAYER

Your base layer sits directly on your skin. On a hot day in the summer it may be just a cotton T-shirt. But in cold weather, the clothing material you put directly against your skin needs to be more carefully chosen. When you are hiking, paddling, or climbing, your body sweats to cool itself. Work hard enough, and you'll sweat profusely even on a winter day. But the minute you stop to rest or when you arrive at camp and quit hiking so hard, you have a layer of water against your skin and the same chilly air outside. The combination of conduction and evaporation under these conditions can cool someone wearing a cotton base layer to a stammering, chattering numbskull in minutes.

A base layer must insulate even when wet and, ideally, wick water away from your skin. Clothing manufacturers have come up with polyester materials that are woven more tightly on the outside of the garment than on the inside. The result is that through capillary action, the water travels from inside to outside faster than through ordinary materials.

My favorite base layer is a very lightweight polyester shirt that has some wicking ability. It's light enough that I can wear it while hiking in warm weather and not get too hot and yet it has all the insulating properties necessary to help keep me warm when the weather gets cold. On cold days, you can use the same type of polyester base layer on your legs.

## INTERMEDIATE LAYERS

The intermediate layers serve as insulation, analogous to the fiberglass baffles in the walls of your house. Their purpose is simply to trap dead air space. You can use polar fleece shirts, pile jackets, wool shirts, down jackets, down vests, or any combination of the lot. I usually use a midweight polyester shirt and a pile jacket for the intermediate layers. If it really gets cold, I'll add a down vest or a down sweater to that combination, provided I'm in a dry climate. In a wet climate I'll add a second pile jacket or wool sweater.

## OUTER LAYER

Your outer layer is just as important as your base layer. The outer layer serves less as an insulator than as a vapor barrier protection against snow, rain, and wind. If you'll suffer through the same building construction analogy, the outer layer is your tin roof. On a windy day, you'll recall, the air circulation can rob your body heat through convection. The best outer layer on a windy day is, not surprisingly, a wind shell or wind jacket. These shells are typically made of a breathable nylon or Gore-Tex. Ounce for ounce, a wind jacket is one of the most effective items for keeping warm on a windy day. I almost always carry a wind jacket or wind shirt, even for short day hikes. It doesn't weigh anything and makes a big, big difference.

On rainy or snowy days, the outer layer needs to be waterproof. You have two basic choices for your outer layer: Gore-Tex or coated nylon. Your choice between the two depends on your budget and on just how wet the conditions are. As noted above, Gore-Tex is the most expensive rain gear, but probably the most versatile. If you can afford the stuff, Gore-Tex clothing makes for a good outer shell.

The most waterproof material is a rubberized nylon, typically worn by fishermen. A heavily rubberized nylon truly is waterproof and that's why fishermen wear the stuff. The obvious disadvantage is that this material, while keeping water out, also keeps water vapor in. So while the rain may not get you, your sweat and steam can soak you, no matter your base layer. Rubberized nylon is most useful for outdoor activities such as rafting, which may involve long periods of sitting in wet conditions.

The ideal outer shell would be a jacket that was totally waterproof and totally breathable. But it doesn't exist. What you gain in waterproofing you lose in breathability. I recommend bringing along two outer layers: a very breathable windbreaker and a waterproof shell of the material of your choice.

## Notes on Clothing Items

**Socks:** If you plan to hike long miles, bring lots of socks. For NOLS courses, we tell students to bring five pairs of wool or synthetic socks. No matter what the length of your trip, you should bring at least three pairs. That way you can wear two pairs and always have a pair of dry socks in the event of an emergency. You can wear wool socks or synthetic socks, but cotton socks have the same disadvantage you would expect from any cotton clothing: They don't keep your feet warm when wet. Fresh socks also help you with your foot care. Socks that have been worn for miles and miles become dirty and crusty and finally abrasive. So keep your socks as clean as you can, wash them frequently, and rotate them in and out of the lineup.

If you haven't hiked much in your boots, consider bringing a pair of thin Capilene or wool socks. Then if your boots are too tight, you can microadjust the fit by wearing the liner socks and a pair of thick socks. If the boots are too large, you can wear the liner socks and two pairs of wool socks.

**Lower body:** On most hiking trips all you need for your lower body are a pair of nylon shorts, a pair of polyester long underwear bottoms or tights, and a pair of wind pants. Nylon shorts make the hot days more tolerable and dry quickly if you swim in them. With nylon shorts, you don't even need to bring underwear. On NOLS courses, we have students bring rugged wind pants with spacious leg room and zippers to allow the pants to be put on and taken off over hiking boots. Wind pants are breathable so you don't get too hot when hiking, yet they serve as good protection against wind and heat loss through convection. Wind pants worn in combination with long underwear bottoms keep you warm at night when in camp or on the coldest trail days.

Long underwear bottoms or tights are great to sleep in, to keep you warm once in camp, or even to hike in when it's very cold. On trips where the temperature might get below freezing, you should consider bringing a second pair of long underwear bottoms or even pile pants.

Some people like to hike in "normal" pants like jeans or cotton khakis. I'm partial to jeans for just about everything from inaugurations to branding cattle, but the truth is they fall short when it comes to hiking, simply because they are pure cotton. If they get wet, they take forever to dry and will conduct your body heat with distressing efficiency. It's akin to wearing copper pants. If you like to hike in "normal" pants, hunt around for a polyester blend either at the thrift shop or at your camping store.

**Camp shoes:** After a long day of hiking, one of the nicest things you can do for yourself is to get out of those huge clunker boots you've worn all day and put on your camp shoes. Camp shoes are simply a pair of lightweight shoes that you can wear around camp or on short day hikes. Tennis shoes with a good tread or light hikers make for the best camp shoes. They are light and still offer enough support or protection to scramble up steep hills, jump streams, etc. Some people bring sandals or Tevas for camp shoes. They're fun and light and comfortable, but they don't protect the feet from sharp rocks or sticks, and if the weather gets very cold so will your feet. Here are some things you should be able to do in your camp shoes: fetch water, go on a five-mile day hike, climb boulders, fish, and pad around camp.

**Gaiters:** Gaiters keep the dirt and pebbles out of your boots and help keep your socks cleaner. Crossing streams, they help keep your feet dry. Wearing gaiters, you're more likely to stay on trails—even muddy ones—and avoid making new ones because the gaiters help keep the water and mud out of your boots.

**Hats:** A warm wool or synthetic hat is one of the most important pieces of clothing you can bring. A pile or wool hat keeps you warm when you sleep or when you summit a peak. You can lose a lot of heat out of your head, so putting a hat on is one of the best and easiest ways to stay warm. The light balaclava is very useful because it can keep your face and neck warm when fully unrolled, or it can be worn as a cap when rolled up. Pound for pound and taking into consideration ease of use, a hat is a great way to regulate your body temperature. Even in the summer, but especially in the spring, fall, and winter, don't forget a warm hat.

A baseball cap or a tennis hat works well to protect your face and head from the sun.

**Gloves:** I bring at least a pair of lightweight wool or polyester gloves on almost every trip. They don't weigh much, and on cold mornings they keep your hands from getting too numb to do the camp chores. Gloves are nice to hike in when you get up high or when the wind picks up. If you're camping in the spring or fall when the weather can lose its composure, a pair of very light liner gloves and a pair of midweight gloves make for a good combination.

## SAVING MONEY ON CLOTHES

Outdoor clothing is expensive. A good storm jacket, with the Gore-Tex and the cachet, costs around $400. A nice pile jacket can run over a hundred dollars. If you bought the most expensive gear at retail prices, you could end up sinking a couple of grand into your clothes alone. So what can you do to economize? In many cases, you can substitute used gear, army surplus gear, or sale gear for the most expensive stuff and still live quite comfortably once you get up into the mountains. For instance, instead of buying a pile jacket, you can use one of your old wool sweaters. Try the army–navy surplus store. They often sell heavy wool shirts that are quite warm. If you know you're going to do a lot of this stuff, you may want to sink some real money into a particularly useful piece of equipment. A storm jacket comes to mind. You can use this for skiing in the winter, mountaineering in the summer, and boating in the fall.

*Figure 4-1 The Economical Wardrobe*

| For the Well-Heeled | Poor Man's Equivalent |
| --- | --- |
| Pile jacket | Wool sweater |
| Gore-Tex shell | Wind shirt |
| Gore-Tex pants | Wind pants |
| Pile pants | Army surplus wool pants |

Sure, some expensive clothing is very well made and very nice to own. But chances are there is a less expensive substitute. The table on page 105 demonstrates the pricey options on the left and the more economical options on the right.

Don't forget that you can borrow clothes—and equipment, for that matter—from your friends. For a one-time raft trip, or a one-time mountaineering trip, when you don't know whether you even like the sport, see if a friend will loan you the gear so you don't have to fork out the big bucks for stuff that may sit in your closet.

# CHAPTER 5

# Camping Technique

Not so long ago an American could ride into a new wilderness, raze a forest, build a cabin, butcher a million buffalo, and perhaps declare statehood. A young nation then, the wilds were for the taking and it seemed to the pioneers that the lands were endless. A mere 200 years later, we have mapped every square foot of the fifty states, covered all but a small portion of the landscape with human "improvements," and brought electricity to nearly every house. The only real frontier left is digital or in space.

But the pioneer spirit hasn't died. Many still go camping with the idea that upon setting foot in the woods they have to conquer something and swing the axe a bit. We have all been in the company of those who, upon arriving in camp, assume the air of Daniel Boone or Davy Crockett, start issuing orders, and produce tools from their pack that would make a carpenter blush. Soon trees are falling, dirt is flying, and flags are planted as these modern-day frontiersmen establish outposts in the wilderness.

They might dig a moat around their tent to channel water in the event of a storm, chop half a cord of firewood, construct some rudimentary furniture, and sink a few nails in the trees to hang utensils. But that is not camping. That is homesteading and, chances are, you're in the company of a novice. The conquest attitude that served our forebears is antithetical to today's wildlands and for today's outdoorsperson. Now, wildlands—the few

*Figure 5-1 Number of Backpackers Age 16 and Older\**

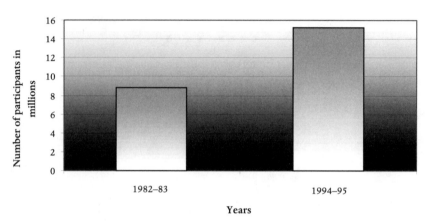

Number of Backpackers

*Source: SMGA and USDA Forest Service, 1977

areas still pristine—are a delicate treasure that needs protecting. If ever the revolutionary motto "Don't tread on me" was apt, it is in reference to these places.

If the aim of the pioneer was to build something that would last a hundred years, the aim of the modern outdoorsperson is to travel through the wilderness leaving no trace of his or her presence. There are simply too many people and too few wildlands left to allow careless travel.

Go to popular recreation areas and they are either very heavily regulated, very heavily damaged from those who camp fortissimo, or both. In some wilderness areas, you need a permit to visit, and land managers decide where you can camp and where you can hike. In other areas you may see fire rings, trees stripped of all their lower branches, assorted trash, human feces, and toilet paper. The garbage and damage is all the uglier when perched in the middle of a pristine natural area.

Even Mount Everest, once the ultimate symbol of the unattainable, is littered with oxygen bottles and garbage from past expeditions trying to get to the summit. The trash heap at the highest camp, just 3,000 feet below the summit, captures the sad side of the human relationship with nature: Entranced by the summit, expeditions scatter Everest with garbage as they attempt to conquer this most prestigious peak.

*Figure 5-2 National Park Recreational Visits 1926–1996\**

**National Park Recreation Visits**

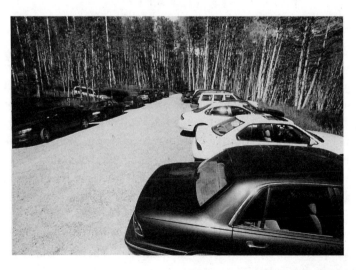

*Source: National Park Service

Camping techniques have dramatically evolved in the last thirty years, as have camping techniques within the NOLS curriculum. As a small example, thirty years ago when Paul Petzoldt started the school, NOLS conservation

The parking lot at a popular trailhead in the Elk Mountains of Colorado. With so many people visiting the backcountry, today's campers have to pay much more attention to their impact than did the campers of yore. *Mark Harvey*

practices—cutting edge at the time—included raging stump fires, and burying empty tin cans under rocks. Actually burying the tin cans was a step
ahead of many campers who merely left the cans in the fire pit. Today, NOLS
courses limit their campfires to small mound fires (discussed later in this
chapter), pitiful (but less damaging) tributes to Petzoldt's glorious bonfires of
the old era, and pack out their trash as well.

This chapter discusses camping techniques used at NOLS. The principles
behind them are simple, safe, and ecologically sound. These camping practices hold true no matter the environment or the activity.

# Choosing a Campsite

At the end of a hard day, the last thing you feel like doing is looking around
for a good campsite. When you're tired, it's tempting to plop your tent down
on the first flat spot you find, no matter the surroundings or the ground surface. But choosing a good campsite is a centerpiece of good camping technique. So when you're done hiking, take your pack off, put on a warm layer
if you feel cold, take a long pull on your water bottle, and eat a snack if you're
low on energy. Then start your search. Remember that great campsites are
found, not made.

### IS IT SAFE?

First and foremost, your campsite must be safe. When you find a potential
site, look around you. Look up. Are you in a climax forest where half the trees
are dead or dying? We call such trees "widow makers" for obvious reasons:
They fall down in windstorms or, failing that, drop huge branches. Are you
below a steep slope covered with loose rocks that could roll down onto your
tent in the night? Are you camped on a ridge top or out in a wide open basin
where lightning is likely to strike? Now look below you. Are you in a seasonal
streambed? If you're in the desert, are you in a gully that will turn into a raging torrent if there is a flash flood? Are you on the edge of a cliff that you'll
forget about when you get up in the night to pee? Are you camped in a basin
that will fill with water if it rains hard? Are you sleeping on a game trail where
big nocturnal animals might stumble over you? If it is winter or spring, are
you in the path of an avalanche? Beach camping? Where is your tent in rela-
tion to the high-tide level?

## Leave No Trace Principles

- ▾ Plan Ahead and Prepare
- ▾ Travel and Camp on Durable Surfaces
- ▾ Dispose of Waste Properly
- ▾ Leave What You Find
- ▾ Minimize Campfire Impacts
- ▾ Respect Wildlife
- ▾ Be Considerate of Other Visitors

# Leave No Trace Camping

In an effort to advance and promote camping practices that have minimum impact on the land, four federal agencies—the Bureau of Land Management, the U.S. Forest Service, the National Park Service, and the U.S. Fish and Wildlife Service—and several private organizations including NOLS have joined together to develop and foster what is called the Leave No Trace (LNT) program. While the LNT program was started in the seventies by the U.S. Forest Service, it is only since the early nineties that it has become accepted as the standard for minimum impact camping techniques in the United States. In 1991, because of its reputation as a leader in minimum impact camping skills and because of the success of Bruce Hampton and David Cole's book, *Soft Paths,* NOLS was asked to develop the educational model for the program. The resulting easy-to-remember principles are used by outdoorspeople in almost all environments.

## 1. PLAN AHEAD AND PREPARE

### Know the Area and What to Expect

By studying the area before you leave on your trip, you will be aware of camping restrictions, fire restrictions, terrain, weather, and the number of visitors using the region. That knowledge will not only help you to choose the most suitable area for your group but will also help you to plan your days so you don't end up late in the evening with no place to camp but a restricted, fragile, or uncomfortable area. Planning ahead improves your chances of making a safe trip and avoiding a costly and intrusive evacuation.

### Equipment

Bringing the proper equipment allows you to camp well. Having warm clothes and a good sleeping bag allows you to stay warm without having to build a big fire. A self-standing tent can be moved easily from site to site in the event that you spend more than one night at the same camp and want to spread out your impact. Good boots and gaiters make it easier and more comfortable to stay on muddy trails—instead of straying off the trails. A trowel makes it easy to bury your feces in a deep cathole.

### Repackage Your Food

Plan your rations carefully to reduce waste and leftovers. Reduce the trash and litter you bring in by repackaging your food into plastic bags and reusable containers.

## 2. TRAVEL AND CAMP ON DURABLE SURFACES

Most environments that we camp and hike in are delicate and need careful handling. Alpine environments have short growing seasons due to thin soils and early winters. In northern Wyoming, for instance, plants have about ninety days to grow before the fall comes. In the desert, plants have little water to sustain them. The woody plants of the forest understory are easily broken by careless footsteps. So when you see a meadow of alpine flowers or a desert environment of cryptobiotic crust, the dark, crusty moss species growing in the southwest desert, remember that growth does not come easily and, damaged, may take years to recover. If you visit the Red Desert in Wyoming, you can still see the ruts made by Americans emigrating west in the 1850s. Though a wonderful historical feature, the ruts illustrate the time it takes for delicate ecologies to recover.

Consider all the activities in the span of one night's stay in the backcountry. You arrive at your site, pitch a tent, establish a place to have a kitchen, get

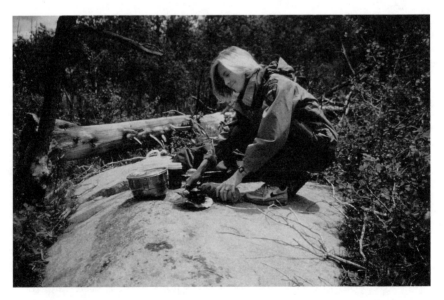

Locating your kitchen on a durable surface—a big rock when possible—is a great way to reduce your impact. *Rich Brame*

water, go to the bathroom, cook dinner, sleep, cook breakfast, pack your things, and finally leave. That twelve-to-sixteen-hour stay includes numerous trips in and out of your camp and using the local water source. How you camp makes a big difference to the environment. If you choose your site carelessly, you'll likely harm the area, whereas if you choose your site carefully, you can camp leaving little trace of your passage.

The ideal surface to camp on is rock. That may sound ridiculously uncomfortable, but the truth is lots of areas have big flat rock surfaces that make wonderful campsites. Whether it's the sandstone of Utah, the granite of Colorado, or the andesite of Washington's Cascades, a rock surface is nearly indestructible and you don't have to worry about damaging the site.

Gravel bars, beaches, snow, and ice are also excellent choices for tent and kitchen sites. You can't do much to hurt the sand and gravel; snow and ice melts or accumulates, obliterating your tracks.

If you can't find a nonvegetated area like the ones above, choose your vegetated site carefully. Studies have shown that dry meadow grasses, sedges, and leaf and needle litter are more durable than, say, the woody plants growing in the forest. Woody plants are tall and broad-leafed to capture the sun. Forbs, herbaceous plants, certain lichens (e.g., foliose and the fruticose), and rotting logs are other delicate features that should be avoided when choosing your campsite.

In general, plants growing in dense mats are also much more hardy than plants growing in isolation. Dry soils are generally more durable than saturated soils.

### Figure 5-3 Camping Surfaces

| Very Durable | Somewhat Durable | Delicate |
|---|---|---|
| Rocks | Dry grass meadows | Forests with woody plants |
| Gravel bars and sandy beaches | Leaf and needle litter | Wet meadows |
| Snowfields and glaciers | Sedges | Sparsely vegetated areas |
| | | Alpine tundra |
| | | Cryptogam |
| | | Lichens |
| | | Forbs and herbaceous plants |

### In Popular Areas, Concentrate Use

The most popular recreation areas often have established campsites where you are required to camp. The reasoning is simple: Concentrating the impact of campers in one small area prevents damaging more pristine sites. The same principles hold true in less traveled areas where there are nevertheless established sites. If you come to the spot where you want to spend the night and you see an obvious campsite—a fire ring and devegetated ground where people have clearly pitched their tents in the past—that is the best place to put your tent and establish your camp. These sites are sometimes called "sacrifice" sites because the damage has already been done. There may be a nicer site nearby which has a superb view and no sign of anyone having camped on it. But if you camp there and the next party that comes along camps there too, soon you will have yet another "sacrifice" area where before there was only one.

### Camp Away from Trails and Water

In most public lands, managers require that you camp at least 200 feet (70 to 80 normal walking steps) from water and trails. Studies show that recreation use right next to water leads to an increase in Giardia contamination and also an adverse effect on aquatic flora and fauna. Camped right next to water, you trample the typically delicate plants growing there and make it harder for wildlife to drink from that particular source.

The regulation prohibiting camping within 200 feet of water and trails also has to do with aesthetics and consideration for others. One of the most unhappy surprises for the person looking to get away from it all comes when she crests a mountain ridge, sees a beautiful lake below, momentarily thinks she has found paradise, and then notices three or four tents pitched right on the lake shore where the views are. It is human to want to camp in the most beautiful sites but also obnoxious. It is akin to climbing onto an opera stage to better hear the soloist, thus diminishing the spectacle for the rest of the audience. That probably sounds windy, but it really is disappointing to find unthoughtful campers camping on the masterpiece.

### In Remote Areas, Spread Use

In pristine areas, it's particularly important to disperse activities and campsites to avoid trampling the vegetation. By taking alternate paths between camp and the water source and the kitchen site, you can avoid excessive trampling and avoid starting new trails. Choosing the most durable surfaces for kitchen sites and tent sites also helps to keep remote sites in their natural state. When you pack up to leave, camouflage and naturalize the area by scattering leaves and twigs and by returning any rocks you may have used to their original locations. At pristine sites, limit your stay to as few nights as possible.

### Avoid Places Where Impact Is Just Beginning

Sometimes an area is neither heavily impacted nor pristine but somewhere in between—it is just beginning to show signs of use. These areas may have matted grass, the beginnings of camp trails, and other signs of human use without being so trampled as to be considered a sacrifice zone. Such places have an excellent chance of recovery if left alone and consequently should be avoided.

### Camp Layout

People spend most of their camp time in the kitchen area. The kitchen becomes the natural focus point of a camp for eating, socializing, and swapping a good yarn. Consequently it gets a lot of traffic. Count the trips in and out of a kitchen—getting water, coming and going for a warm layer, fishing for a snack, etc.—and consider the activity in the kitchen—cooking, washing dishes—and you can well imagine your kitchen site getting hammered by hard use. On NOLS courses, we go to extra lengths to locate our kitchens on surfaces that can take a pounding. As with your campsite, the best kitchen location is a flat rock or a sandy area. If you can't find such durable surfaces, dry meadow grass, sedges, or litter is your next best choice.

The area around your pack also gets hit hard from trips to and fro fetching clothing, food, and gear. The area least impacted is usually around your tent—the sleeping area. The best layout in a pristine area is to make three separate sites: one for your kitchen, one for your pack, and one for your tent. Vary your path among the three sites so you don't create trails.

## 3. DISPOSE OF WASTE PROPERLY

### Pack It In Pack It Out

This is a simple rule. Pack out any garbage that you generate, organic or otherwise. When fishing, pick up your stray fishing line so waterfowl don't tangle themselves in it. When cooking, pick up spilled food scraps so you don't attract critters or leave an unsightly mess for the next people who come along. Pack out leftovers instead of scattering them so animals don't become habituated to people and their food. Watch for the little wrappers on gum and candy. Even "micro" trash degrades the environment and accumulates over the years.

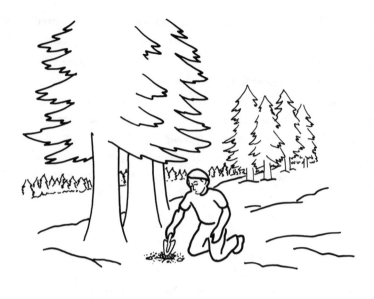

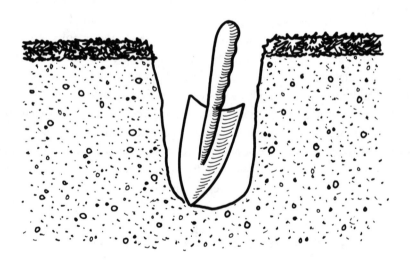

Human feces should be buried in a "cathole" 6 to 8 inches deep and at least 200 feet away from water.

Keeping a tight and tidy camp will keep the wind from scattering your garbage and scraps to the four corners of the globe.

### Human Waste

Human feces have little nice to recommend them, especially in the back-country. If you want to learn how to dispose of your human waste properly, study your Siamese or tabby cat and watch what they do. They find the best location, their litter box; they dig a shallow hole, evacuate themselves, bury what they bore, and get on with the day. They do this all with a grace and cleanliness that outdoorspeople should strive for. Take your other pet, your dog, and watch him. He's of the old school and needs to learn something from your cat. He'll run outside and squat unceremoniously wherever he pleases, leaving you a treasure you'll most likely find with your new suede shoes. Crude, you say? Well, Homo sapiens in some cases are no better. Many campsites are covered with toilet paper and feces a scant few yards from the established tent site. One of the most important camping techniques to know is, to put it delicately, how to defecate properly in the woods. Since the mountains don't have litter boxes, you'll have to choose the best place to bury your fecal waste. The principles are simple.

### Avoid Polluting Water Sources

Human feces are loaded with pathogens and if we defecate near water, whatever pathogens are present in our feces are eventually introduced to the nearest water source. Water sources include not only lakes, rivers, and streams, but also areas that will carry a runoff (e.g., dry streambeds and gullies). So, as a rule of thumb, take your dump at least 200 feet from water sources.

### Avoid Contact with Insects and Animals

Feces left to decompose on the surface make attractive targets for animals and insects. Animals and insects ingest the feces and become, in the parlance of epidemiologists, disease vectors. That simply means the animals and insects who ingest our feces and hence our pathogens travel throughout the wilds spreading those same pathogens. Not only will the animals spread the pathogens, but they themselves may suffer from them as well.

### Maximize Decomposition

Find an environment that will help to decompose your feces. Recent studies show that it can take a year or more for human waste to decompose in the outback. Feces decompose most efficiently in organic soil, which is soil loaded with microorganisms. Organic soil is usually dark and rich-looking. By contrast, mineral soil is sandy and rocky and doesn't have the rich dark color of organic soil. Mineral soil lacks the abundance of microorganisms necessary to decompose feces.

### Minimize the Chances of Social Impact

Once you find a good spot that meets the criteria listed above, dig a cathole about 6 to 8 inches deep with your trowel, a stick, or your boot heel. Do

your business in the small hole and then fill it in using the same dirt you excavated. Out of consideration for your campmates and for sanitation reasons,
your trowel should not touch the human waste during any of this process.
Disguise the area with branches, leaves, pine needles, etc., before you leave.

Most people choose to bring toilet paper on their trips. If you do bring it,
the best way to dispose of it is to pack it out in a plastic bag. If buried, the toilet paper is slow to decompose and animals usually dig it up in the meantime.
In addition, toilet paper is difficult to burn completely and there are docu-
mented cases of even experienced campers lighting the woods on fire as they
try to burn their used toilet paper.

Consider not bringing toilet paper at all. There are lots of natural alternatives out there such as moss, smooth rocks, sticks, and snow.

### Bathing

Good sanitation is essential in the outdoors, and on long trips that may include bathing. If you bathe on your camping trip, go easy on the soap—even
if it is biodegradable—and use it at least 200 feet away from water sources.
Soap changes the aquatic biology and can harm plants, animals, and fish. If
you use soap for washing your body or your clothes, use cooking pots and
collapsible water jugs to haul water at least 70 paces from the lake or stream.

## 4. LEAVE WHAT YOU FIND

### Minimize Site Alterations

In the old days of camping, men and women didn't hesitate to alter their
sites with spade work that would make the Bureau of Reclamation envious.
The new ethic of camping calls for you to leave your site as undisturbed as
you found it. Instead of digging a drainage moat around your tent, it's better
to find a site that drains naturally. Not only will you do less harm to the area
but you'll likely stay drier as well. Instead of reworking a site—moving great
boulders and ripping out vegetation—to make it more comfortable, hunt
around a bit and you'll likely find a comfortable spot to sleep that needs no
improvement. Having a decent sleeping pad helps here as well. If you need
to move a rock to stake down your tent, put it back in the hole where you
found it so the site looks natural when you leave.

### Avoid Damaging Live Trees and Plants

Except in emergencies (being separated from your tent, perhaps), you
should be able to camp comfortably without harming the trees and plants at
your site. If you tie your tent lines to a tree, pick a decent-sized one so it sur-

vives the use. Cutting tree boughs for extra padding under your sleeping bag is an obsolete technique; it's something for the survival situation when you have to spend a night out without your sleeping gear.

### Leave Natural and Cultural Artifacts

When you stumble upon the perfect arrowhead, eagle feather, or geode, it's only human to want to bring it home for your mantelpiece. But the wild areas are a sort of museum of cultural and natural history and if we all take home souvenirs, pretty soon all those interesting parts are gone. What's more, removing natural objects or excavating archaeological, cultural, and historical artifacts from any public land is prohibited under the Archaeological Resources Protection Act of 1979 and the National Historic Preservation Act of 1966.

## 5. MINIMIZE CAMPFIRE IMPACTS

Fires are fun and in some ways capture the essence of camping. They offer a center point and a sense of hearth even miles out of town. When the conversation comes to a grinding halt, you can just watch the log pop and crack. What's more primitive, comforting, and pleasing than a fire deep into a cool night?

Now let me spoil all that by saying the modern outdoorsperson limits his use of fires in the backcountry because there isn't necessarily enough wood for all the campers to have fires every night. Have you ever been to a popular campsite that has all the trees stripped of their branches, and its ground picked clean of dead wood? The camp feels as if it has been looted and even if you have the entire campsite to yourself, the bald trees bring back the dog-eat-dog, economically shortaged world you tried to leave behind. What's more, collecting and burning all the dead wood will make the soil poorer. Decomposing wood is a compost to the soil and adds elements such as carbon and nitrogen, which help plants grow.

The other problem with fires—at least those built the old-fashioned way— is that they leave unsightly scars of blackened rock and torched vegetation. What's more, the fire of yore often ended up becoming a garbage receptacle. Fires in and of themselves aren't antithetical to the wilderness ethic; but fires built in the wrong place, built carelessly, and fire sites that end up as trash receptacles fly in the face of modern camping technique.

When the weather conditions are right and there's plenty of wood, you can build a fire and have little impact on the environment given the right techniques.

### Be Aware of Regulations and Weather Conditions

Land managers prohibit building fires in hot, dry conditions when the chance of starting a forest fire is high. They also prohibit fires in very heavily used areas where there is little firewood available. Fires are usually banned above the treeline because wood is scarce. Check on fire regulations before hitting the trail. Even when fires are permitted, make your own judgment of the hazards based on wind conditions and the condition of the plants around you. A windy day, a dry understory, and an errant spark . . . the inferno.

### Use Dead and Downed Wood—Small in Size

How do you know if there's enough wood in the area for your fire? There's no scientific answer to that question, but if you have to hunt very hard to get an armload of sticks, chances are there is too little wood in the area. And if taking an armload of wood makes a noticeable difference in how the landscape looks, there's too little wood as well.

Studies have shown that the leaves, major branches, and trunks of decomposing trees add nitrogen and carbon to the soils. Thus burning major logs and branches robs soils of important parts in the nutrient cycle. Small branches, on the other hand, are less important in replenishing soils. That's one good reason to burn small branches in your fire instead of the mighty Yule logs. Another reason not to burn the big dead logs is that they make homes for certain birds and animals, and act as check dams against sheet erosion. Finally, when it comes to aesthetics, an area stripped of all its big snags and downed logs loses its wild quality.

It should be obvious why you burn dead wood—green wood doesn't burn worth a hoot. The reason for burning downed wood has to do with aesthetics. Breaking branches off dead trees and chopping down dead trees is the calling card of a heavy-handed camper.

When you do hunt for wood, walk out of your camp five or ten minutes and get it from a broad area so as to spread out your impact.

### Care and Feeding of Your Fire

Keep a trowel or vessel of water near your fire in case it catches the nearby vegetation. Burn your fire down to the ash so you don't leave blackened stubs on the site. This takes more time but makes a difference in reducing signs of your fire. If you have extra wood left after you've finished with your fire, scatter it around. Leaving wood for the next camper, while it may seem a nice courtesy, encourages the use of fire and takes away from any pristine quality the spot may have possessed.

## Cleaning Up

Douse your fire with water before leaving camp and check the ashes for hot cinders. Scatter the cooled ashes over a wide area and they will soon blend into the environment. If you use an existing fire ring, try to make it as attractive as possible for the next campers so they will use the same ring.

## Use Existing Fire Rings

If you're camping in a popular recreation area, you will likely find existing fire rings almost everywhere. It makes no sense ecologically or otherwise to build a new ring. It also doesn't make sense to dismantle the rings in heavy-use areas when you leave camp because the next people to come along will probably build a new one.

## Use LNT Fire-Building Techniques

In the old days, if you wanted a fire, you simply gathered about twenty rocks, made a small ring in the most convenient location, gathered wood from the nearest trees, lit a match, and kicked back next to the flames. The problem with the old way is that the fire scorched and sterilized the ground underneath it as well as blackened the rocks. To reduce this damage, someone invented pit fires. Pit fires are built by digging out a piece of sod, building your fire on the mineral soil, and then replacing the sod when you are done. But pit fire sites sink after time and leave obvious signs behind them. Now, we have better techniques for building fires in pristine areas.

## Portable Fire Pans

Fire pans are metal containers with three-inch or higher sides to contain the ashes. River guides have used them for years and today backpackers and horsepackers are using them as well. You can buy a commercial fire pan or improvise with a garbage can lid or oil pan. With fire pans, you simply locate your pan on a durable surface such as rock or a gravel bed, fill the pan with mineral soil, have your fire, and disperse the ashes when you're done. If you can't find a durable surface, you can suspend your fire pan with small boulders.

## Building a Fire on a Gravel or Sand Bar

A good, easy place to build a fire, when you're camped near a river or by the ocean, is on a sand or gravel bar below the high-water line. Make a small pit to contain the fire and build it right on the sand or gravel. When the fire is out completely, scatter the doused ashes and fill in the pit with the same material you dug out. The next high water will wash away whatever remains are left of your fire. Note that it can be some time between floods, so don't leave ashes and charcoal where they can be seen. Even if you build your fire on a sand or gravel bar, you should still camp at least 200 feet from the water.

## Mound Fires

The nice thing about mound fires is that you can build them on a variety of ground surfaces from rock to leaf litter without damaging the ground. The mound, if made thick enough, insulates the ground from the fire.

To build a mound fire, grab your trowel and gather about two large stuff sacks of mineral soil (you can turn your stuff sack inside out to keep the inside from getting dirty). Mineral soil is like sand or gravel: It does not have the rich organic content of fertile soil. You find mineral soil in streambeds and from the holes left by recently uprooted trees.

To make cleanup easy, put a fire blanket or ground cloth folded in quarters directly on the spot. Spread the mineral soil on the blanket or ground cloth in a mound about 18 to 24 inches in diameter and about 6 to 8 inches deep (to insulate the ground and the ground cloth). Make a small rim in the soil on the outside of the mound to keep the ashes and cinders from rolling off. If you use a ground cloth, make sure it is entirely covered with soil so you don't burn holes into it.

Build your fire right on the mineral soil. Cleaning up a mound fire is easy: Once you have doused and scattered the ashes, simply pick up the ground cloth with all the mineral soil and return it to the place (river or downed tree cavity) where you got it.

## To Start a Fire

Fire building is an art, but a simple art that shouldn't be shrouded behind too much of the rugged mountain-man mystique. Fledgling arsonists often make the mistake of trying to start a fire with poor wood or not enough small wood to keep the fire going. They light the fire, have it flare up briefly, and then run out of wood. Or they don't gather enough small wood and try, futilely, to light behemoth branches. The best fire builders I know spend a good deal of time preparing the fire before lighting a match. They take the time to collect good, dry kindling so they can build a decent structure and keep the thing going once lit.

A fire needs three things: fuel, oxygen, and ignition. Your fuel needs to be small and dry when you start the fire. Look under ledges, rocks, and at the base of trees. If it doesn't snap smartly when you break it, it's probably wet or green. You can use your knife to make shavings, which light like paper. Your fire needs good airflow when you light it and once it's burning. Some

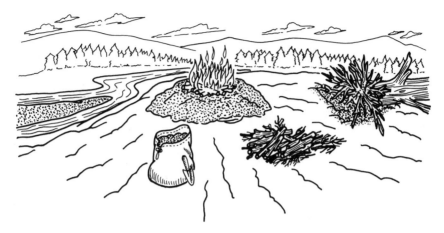

The mound fire is a good way to have a campfire without leaving a blackened fire ring and burning the vegetation. Look on gravel bars and in the cavities left by fallen trees for mineral soil.

## Fire-Starting Tips

▾ Collect enough small dry wood to easily light and feed your fire once lit.

▾ Build your fire in a protected area (behind a rock or bush, for instance). It will be easier to light and less likely to spread if a wind gust hits you.

▾ Build a teepee or log cabin–like structure out of the kindling so the fire has plenty of airflow.

▾ If the wood is wet or green and you need a fire for an emergency, soak twigs in your gas bottle for a good fire starter.

people build a teepee-like structure to allow airflow, others construct small log cabins or lean-tos. You can build any variation of these structures as long as they allow good airflow.

As an outdoorsperson, you should become comfortable with fires in case you need one in an emergency. Knowing how to build a fire may save your life in a tight situation. If you someday find yourself without shelter on a cold night, building a fire may be what saves you from hypothermia. Should your stove fail, knowing how to build and cook on a fire will allow you to eat warm meals.

## 6. RESPECT WILDLIFE

If, as described in the Wilderness Act, we are just "visitors" to the wild areas, then it is our job to treat the wild residents with respect. Wild animals live on the margins when it comes to food and nutrition so any disturbances make their survival that much harder. A deer made to run great distances because of human presence will dip into its energy reserves and stress its entire organism. A calving elk has a hard enough job without being harassed—even if unintentionally—by the eager photographer.

Unleashed dogs are particularly hard on wildlife for obvious reasons: They love a good chase and in the worst cases manage to kill what they're after.

Feeding animals, while it may seem an act of kindness, does the animals no good. It habituates them to humans and can make them dependent on handouts.

## 7. BE CONSIDERATE OF OTHER VISITORS

When you take the time and effort to get away to the outback you probably had some peace and quiet in mind. Most people do. Probably the biggest social impact you can make is with loud noise, either shouting or with electronic devices like radios. There is nothing quite so obnoxious as settling in for a nice evening dinner only to have your reverie broken by your camp neighbors shouting back and forth to each other. Respect others' privacy and their right to some peace.

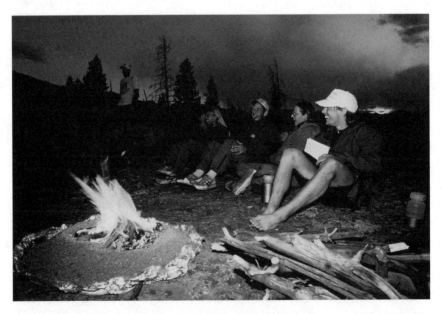

NOLS students enjoying the heat and atmosphere of a low-impact mound fire. By building the fire on gathered mineral soil and by using small dead and downed wood, a mound fire leaves little trace on the environment. *John McConnell*

# Bear Camping

Both grizzly and black bears are omnivores, very clever, and nearly prehensile. They have an exquisite sense of smell and nothing will tempt them more than pan-fried trout, margarine, and the smell of your pancakes in the morning. The reason to practice special bear-camping techniques is not just for your own safety, but for the safety of the bears as well. The easier it is for a bear to get human food, the more habituated it becomes to humans, up to the point where it has no fear of entering a camp to get what it pleases. It becomes a "problem bear" and eventually will be shot by land managers if it ransacks one too many camps. Where I live, wildlife agents have a bear policy of "two strikes and you're out." If a bear causes trouble—raiding garbage cans, entering a house, etc.—twice, a wildlife agent will shoot it. This month alone, in the county where I live, land managers have shot five black bears who have been too tempted by the smell of human garbage or barbecue grills. When you think about it, we are considerably more dangerous to bears than they are to us. According to Steven Herrero, a preeminent bear expert, there were fewer than 200 grizzly-related injuries between 1900 and 1980, and only 14 deaths. While black bears have attacked humans hundreds of times, of the 500 people attacked between 1960 and 1980, 90 percent of the injuries were considered minor. I am not suggesting that these animals can be cuddled. Threatened or enraged, they are dangerous and sometimes deadly.

There are three species of bears in North America: black bears, grizzly bears, and polar bears. Black bears are by far the most common. In the lower 48 states, there are roughly ten times as many black bears as grizzly bears. In fact, only about 1,000 grizzly bears are left in the lower 48 states. What's more, black bears are distributed throughout much of the continental United States from Maine to California while grizzlies are only found in the northwestern states of Wyoming, Montana, Idaho, and Alaska. Polar bears inhabit only the very northern climes, are the largest of the bear species, and arguably the most dangerous to humans. We will limit our discussion here to black and grizzly bears.

Black bears are smaller than grizzly bears and, having evolved in the wooded mountains, generally respond to danger by fleeing and/or climbing a tree. Grizzly bears evolved out in the open spaces—the plains and the tundra—and thus their response to danger can be aggressive. A grizzly bear's response to humans is less predictable than that of a black bear.

## Bear Camping Basics

▼ Conscientious bear camping is just as important to survival of bears as it is to our own safety. Letting bears get at your food habituates them to humans and makes them "problem bears."

▼ Keep an eye out for signs of bears. Look for scat, tracks, and good bear habitat. Bear habitat has lots of berries, grubs, fish, and carrion.

▼ Avoid surprising bears in dense forests or brush by making plenty of noise as you move up the trail.

▼ Keep your kitchen separate from your campsite. Keep food smells off your person by not wiping your face or clothes with your hands when cooking.

▼ Build a good bear hang at least 10 feet off the ground and at least 4 feet from the nearest branch. Hang all your food and odorous things—toothpaste, soap, and utensils—in the hang.

▼ If charged by a bear, hold your ground and don't run. When in a group of four or more, bunch together and expand your presence by waving your arms and speaking to the bear in a firm tone.

▼ If attacked by a grizzly, play dead and try to get on your stomach with your legs spread. If attacked by a black bear, fight back fiercely.

## WHERE THE BEARS ARE

If you know where bears live, what they like to eat, and the seasons they inhabit the various areas you're visiting, you have a better chance of avoiding a nasty confrontation. Bear tracks are easy to distinguish from, say, canine tracks both by their size and shape. Bear scat also stands apart from other animals because of the size of the diameter and the mixed contents ranging from seeds to animal hair. In addition to scat and tracks, keep your eyes open for fresh claw marks on trees, upturned rocks, and disturbed, rotten stumps. Consult a text on North American mammals to familiarize yourself with bear signs.

Bears eat a wide variety of things including berries, grubs, small animals, fish, and carrion. Keeping your eyes open for bear food will help alert you to the possibilities of bears in the area. A meadow with acres of ripe berries, a rotting elk carcass, and a fish stream meandering through it would be a nice place for a bear to gorge itself. Anytime you smell the odor of carrion in bear country, you should be wary of an encounter: They are attracted by the smell of an animal carcass. Walking through a meadow of anthills and tender plants such as fireweed, keep your eyes open for a bear feeding.

Most bears will avoid you if they can. But a surprised bear—a bear approached unawares—might attack out of a sense of endangerment. Your job as a hiker or camper in bear country is to let a bear know you're in the area and avoid surprising it. In bear country, when crossing areas of dense brush or thick forest, make some noise—

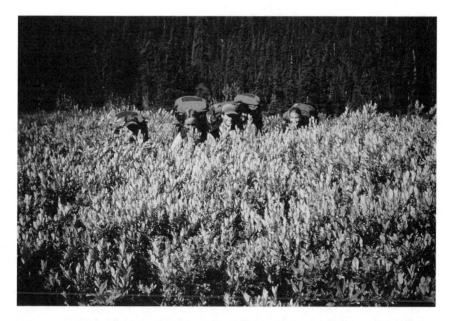

When you are crossing bear habitat with thick brush, the limited visibility makes it easy to surprise a bear. Let the bears know you're in the area by making some noise—talk, sing, or bang a pan. *NOLS Library*

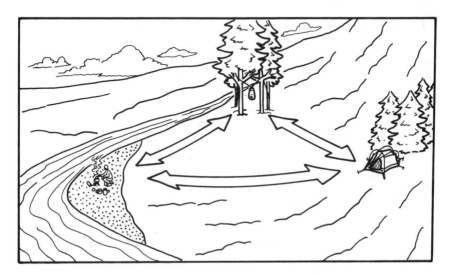

In bear country, locate your kitchen near water on a sandbar, if possible. Locate your tent at least 100 yards away from your kitchen, preferably uphill and upwind. Hang food at least 100 yards from camp.

talk, sing, bang a pan—so a bear bedded down for the day or a bear distracted by a grub bonanza knows you're coming. Take into account the visibility you have in front of you, the wind direction, and the surrounding noise of, say, a large river. All these factors help determine whether or not a bear will know you're coming.

## YOUR CAMPSITE
## IN BEAR COUNTRY

Once in camp, the smells of your rations and wonderful cooking will certainly interest and perhaps tempt bears in the nearby area. Consequently, you should take certain precautions to keep from tempting the hungry creatures too terribly. You can use some strategic layouts for your camp to give yourself the best chance of avoiding bears. The kitchen site goes down on a gravel bar next to the stream or river. If you don't have a gravel bar, cook in an open meadow so you have some visibility. Your tent should be at least 100 yards from your kitchen site. Ideally your tent will be uphill and upwind from your kitchen so the descending air currents do not bring food smells into your camp.

It's important that you concentrate your food smells at the kitchen and not at your tent. In areas where you have sighted bears, you may even want to cook in your wind pants and wind shirt and then leave those clothes with your food at night. You can reduce the food odors by digging a small sump hole (6 to 12 inches deep) and using it to dump your dirty dish water, soapy water, and toothpaste spit. Try not to wipe your face and clothes with your hands while cooking or you have in a way seasoned yourself for consumption. Fish are very strong-smelling and tempting to bears. If you fish for your dinner, throw the viscera in the stream or lake so it's less odorous. If the backcountry has obvious and fresh bear sign, you may just forgo the fishing.

## BEAR HANGS

Unless you camp in a treeless area such as Alaska's tundra country, hanging your food at night in bear country is necessary and in some instances mandated by law. Everything with any sort of appetizing odor should be hung with your food in one of these bear hangs including toothpaste, soap, kitchen utensils, and garbage. Bear hangs should be at least 100 yards from your campsite and preferably downwind. Agency laws require that you hang your food at least 10 feet above the ground and at least 4 feet from the nearest tree branch or tree trunk. Don't underestimate the agility and inventiveness of bears. They have managed to ransack some of my best efforts at a good hang.

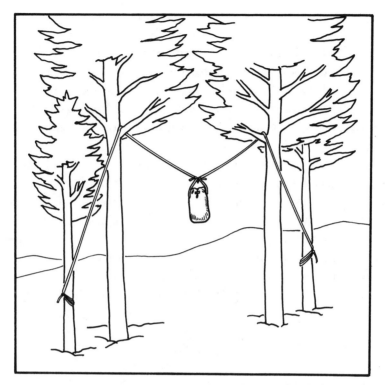

Every tree configuration is different and sometimes you have to use your imagination building a bear hang. Hang food at least 10 feet off the ground and at least 4 feet from the nearest branch or trunk.

I once hung food from near the top of a sharply leaning pine tree, certain that the bear would have no chance at getting the food. The bag was easily 15 feet from the ground, and 10 feet from the tree itself. I slept soundly that night certain that no bear would have a chance at my food. A surprise awaited me in the morning. When I went to get coffee from my hang, a mother bear had climbed the neighboring tree, bent it with her weight, and was playing an Ursus version of piñata-cum-tetherball with my prized food. Meanwhile, her cub gorged itself at the base of the tree with the booty falling all about it. The coffee had to wait.

The basic equipment for a bear hang includes two 40- to 60-foot pieces of 6 millimeter perlon rope (or rope of the equivalent strength), 2 to 3 carabiners (to attach bags or make pulley systems), a 9-inch piece of 1-inch nylon webbing, and a small stuff sack. It's not easy to get 10 or 20 or 30 pounds of food suspended in the air out of reach of a bear. In fact, it can be downright maddening when you don't have a good tree or a good angle or a good technique. The ideal site for a bear hang is arguably a stout branch of a tree 15 or more feet off the ground, without too many small branches in the way. If you find such a branch, you can attach the stuff sack (filled with small rocks for throwing weight) to one end of the rope, toss the rope end over the branch, tie it to your food bag with a bowline knot, and then haul up your food bag by pulling on the other end of the rope. Tie off the rope with friction wraps around a nearby tree.

If you can't find such an ideal branch or if you have several food bags, you may have to use two trees. You can use either a stout branch on each tree or the crotch where the trunk splits. Throw one rope over each tree and then join each rope to your food bag. Raise the bag by pulling the other ends of each rope and tie off with friction wraps. A variation of this, if you have several bags, is to tie the ropes to each other and then tie various butterfly knots along them, where you can attach individual food bags.

In some cases, you may find a tree with such good, solid branches that climbing it may be your best option for building a bear hang. But be sure that the tree really is safely climbable—it's likely that more people are injured from building bear hangs than they are from bear bites.

### When There Are No Trees for a Bear Hang

In places where there are no trees to hang your food—in parts of Alaska, for instance—land managers may require you to store your food in special bear-resistant canisters. Commercially manufactured canisters are made of aluminum or special plastic and range in size from roughly 500 cubic inches to 1,000 cubic inches. They cost between $70 and $200. If you don't use a canister, store your food on the ground at least 100 yards from your tent or sleeping area. Storing your food in a nylon zip bag lined with a large garbage bag helps reduce the food odors.

## ENCOUNTERING A BEAR

If all goes well, your encounters with a bear will be at a comfortable distance of several hundred yards. Should that be the case, quietly move off in a direction away from the bear or allow the bear to move away from you. If you encounter a bear at a distance of less than 100 yards, let it know of your presence with a low, firm voice and by waving your arms. Avoid showing signs of aggression, which include making eye contact and moving toward the bear. When in a group of four or more, bunch together and wave your arms.

## Pepper Sprays

▾ Pepper sprays are made from capsicum (tropical pepper plants) and have proven to be one of the most effective deterrents to an attacking bear.

▾ Pepper sprays must be accessible. No pepper spray will help you if it's buried in your backpack. Keep the spray on your hipbelt or sternum strap.

▾ Practice drawing and firing the pepper spray before you go into bear country to familiarize yourself with the action.

▾ If attacked, aim for the bear's face. The spray won't deter the bear unless it hits it squarely in the face.

▾ Sprays have an effective range of only 10 to 15 feet.

▾ The pepper sprays are actually tasty to bears, and studies show that once sprayed on the ground, they attract bears.

▾ Don't become a sloppy camper and traveler just because you have a pepper spray. It is far better to avoid a confrontation with a bear than to find yourself in a position where you have to use the spray.

Bears, with their poor eyesight, may interpret groups of people to be one large animal.

In the unhappy event of a charging bear, do not run. Most charges are bluffs meant to intimidate, but a fleeing person can excite a bear to a full attack. If you are alone, stand your ground and be quiet. When in a group of four or more, stand together, wave your arms, and speak to the bear in a firm voice. In either case, if the bear comes within spraying distance—and you're carrying pepper spray—aim for the bear's face and shoot in short blasts.

## IF ATTACKED

If a bear actually attacks you, your response depends on the species. With grizzly bears, because they are so powerful, your best response is to play dead. If possible lie on your stomach with your feet spread apart (this makes it harder for the bear to flip you over and attack your face), cover the back of your neck with your hands, and if you're wearing a backpack, leave it on for added protection. Studies have shown that you should wait until the bear actually attacks before you play dead. Otherwise, dropping to the ground may turn what might otherwise have been a bluff charge into a mauling. Most victims who played dead in a grizzly attack have survived without serious injuries. The bear usually bites or swats a few times and leaves. Make sure it has really left before you get up again.

Most experts say you should defend yourself aggressively if attacked by a black bear. They are smaller and you have a fighting chance to fend one off. Use your hands, any available weapon and the pepper spray if you have it.

# On Good Habits

Camping well involves good habits perhaps even more than skill. If you get in the habit of always windproofing your camp, you will not lose important items (such as your wind pants) to the wind. NOLS courses spend the first few days camping very deliberately. They might analyze a site as a group, noting its advantages and disadvantages. Upon leaving camp they sometimes do group "camp checks" to look for items left behind and to take note of the damage done to a site or, ideally, the little trace left by camping mindfully.

It can seem remedial to camp so deliberately. In print it looks insultingly elementary. But professionals and artists who excel in their craft usually master the basics to the point that they don't have to think about them. Soldiers learn to assemble and disassemble weapons blindfolded, sailors tie knots and rig their boats almost unconsciously. Paul Petzoldt says that it is good camping practices that make or break many big expeditions.

Mastering the basics and developing good habits goes a long way. Pack the organized pack, pitch the tight tent, windproof your camp, practice good hygiene, stay hydrated, and eat well. In doing so, you will reduce the chances of injury and sickness, losing equipment, and will probably enjoy your trip.

Small mistakes can snowball into trip-ending disasters. Let's say you pitch your tent poorly—don't anchor it well with the parachute cord—and choose an unprotected site. During the night a 50 mph wind buffets your camp and shreds your tent. Even if you repair the tent, it will not have the same strength it had before. Now you will put yourself in danger if you try to complete the high route along the windy mountains. Had you taken the time to pitch your tent well, you would have been sitting pretty.

Bombproof camping habits are the foundation of good outdoorsmanship. Build, maintain, and constantly improve your foundation of consistent habits.

If this chapter sounds like a manual on how to gut the fun from your camping trips—no big fires, no camping on the nice spots, no sudsing up in the pristine lakes—perhaps you are thinking this is camping for puritans. But your camping needn't be disagreeable or ungainly. Besides, all the threats and admonitions in the world can't change the way you camp over the long run. Ultimately you are out there on your own and will have to make these decisions for yourself. In some ways, the care required to camp well flies in the face of the freedom the outdoors presents. The direction of camping technique today at the turn of the millennium resembles the direction hunting has taken. Once upon a time when this country was thick with game and sparsely populated you could hunt what you wanted, when you wanted, and how many you wanted. But the population grows and the number of wild areas shrinks or remains fixed in the best of circumstances. Hunters have had to adjust to short hunting seasons with strict regulations. As more and more people head to the wildlands and "love them to death," land managers are forced to order more restrictions and regulations. How much they have to restrict regulations probably depends just as much on *how* people camp as on how many people camp.

Eventually you will have to develop your own outdoor ethic and decide how you want to camp. But the fact is we all do have to work a little harder to camp well so that the few wilds remaining stay wild.

# CHAPTER 6

# Travel Technique

W hat makes a good backcountry traveler? To answer that question, it might be instructive to consider some of the best backcountry travelers in human history: the Native American Indians. In a desperate—and ultimately futile—attempt to escape the U.S. cavalry, the Nez Percé Indians traveled upwards of 40 miles a day through the roughest country imaginable in 1877. In a wonderful book titled *Children of Grace*, Bruce Hampton describes the plight of the Nez Percé as they outwitted and out-traveled the U.S. cavalry for several months and over several hundred miles of country. Despite traveling with infants, aged, and the ill, the Nez Percé crossed great rivers, hunted game, stole horses, negotiated steep valleys and passes, left scant signs of their passage, and navigated brilliantly to stay just a step ahead of the government soldiers. So efficient and so clever were the Nez Percé that their efforts caused one particularly hardened soldier to concede, "I am actually beginning to admire their bravery and their endurance in the face of so many well-equipped enemies."*

*Children of Grace* is a terribly sad story, but reading it, I felt the same thing the soldier felt: keen admiration for their mastery of travel in the wilderness. Certainly that mastery came of living in the wilderness day in and day out

---

*Bruce Hampton, *Children of Grace*, Henry Holt and Company, 1994, p. 270.

and few of us will ever approach their level of competence. But some modern men and women who spend a lot of time in the backcountry learn to be remarkably capable travelers. We're not talking brute force here. We're not talking about humping a pack 30 miles without breaking a sweat (or suffering a thought). Certainly it does help to be strong, but intelligence, highly developed skills, and, pardon me here, judgment born of experience or using your brain, go further than the heroic power of a triathlete.

So what does it take to be a really good backcountry traveler? You have to know how to conserve energy, how to feed and hydrate your body, how to navigate, how to read the terrain and know what's really dangerous versus merely tricky, and how to keep your and your group's morale running high. Most any reasonably intelligent person with the desire to learn those things can. But learning those skills takes some time, thought, and even reflection. The novice sets out to cross a patch of hard-featured terrain and, upon encountering a steep, shaley, exposed slope—far more treacherous than anything he has ever crossed—sensibly turns around. The question is planted in his head: What terrain can I safely cross and what terrain is beyond my skills? The smart novice will seek tutorship from—who knows—his local mountain club, a mountaineering course, or just an experienced friend. Armed with more knowledge and experience, he comes upon similar terrain on a later trip, and now crosses it, still within his comfort level, or perhaps turns around again but this time more sure of his decision. This conservative approach in the backcountry may be construed as too cautious or, worse, cowardly, but that's how some of the best mountaineers in the world learned their art. Patiently developing their skills, they reach the level where they can comfortably cross terrain that was once truly hairy to them.

Every time you get a little lost, underestimate the distance on your map, manage to keep your shelter up in a raging storm—every time you manage those setbacks without maiming yourself or the friends traveling with you, you become a better traveler. But it is an art or a skill that only comes with time spent in the backcountry.

## Energy Conservation, Hydration, and Nutrition

If you have never carried a heavy pack over difficult terrain, you may be surprised at how exhausting it is the first couple of days. People new to backpacking struggle with balancing heavy loads, using new muscles they never knew they had, and adjusting to the discomfort of a pack. Even veterans suffer the first few days if they have had too easy a winter. You can make your life easier by practicing energy conservation techniques, staying hydrated, and feeding yourself frequently.

## PACE

Novices to the backcountry often make one of two mistakes. The ambitious ones leave the roadhead like a shot and race up the trail only to exhaust themselves shortly into the day. The ones in poor physical condition slog along the trail and stop for long and frequent breaks. Neither approach leads to efficient backcountry travel. Walk at a steady pace all day, taking short rest breaks at regular intervals, and in the long run you can travel more miles with fewer injuries than if you go trucking across the hills in a hurry.

How fast we travel in the backcountry depends on the fitness level of the entire group, the terrain, the altitude, and our pack weight. But we will be most efficient if we choose a pace that the entire group can maintain comfortably for hours. One of the best ways to measure and regulate your pace is to pay close attention to the tempo of your breathing. The idea is that your breathing should determine your pace, not the other way around. Paul Petzoldt likens it to keeping your engine running at the same RPMs all day, no matter the terrain. On level ground, let's say you take three steps per inhalation and three steps per exhalation. Climbing a hill, while maintaining the same breathing rate, your steps per inhalation may fall to two or even one. At very high altitudes on steep terrain, your pace may slow to several breaths per step.

A good rule of thumb is to hike at a pace slow enough so that you can carry on a conversation (if a breathless one going up hills). Hiking is an aerobic sport and you want to keep your heart rate at an aerobic level (below 150 beats per minute). Since you'll resemble the proverbial tortoise carrying your pack anyway, you might as well travel like the tortoise, not the profligate hare.

Keep in mind the time you'll be spending in the mountains. Perhaps you can afford to exhaust yourself if you're only going on an overnight trip, but if you plan something longer than three days, you will need energy later on. If you hike too hard the first couple of days, you run the risk of injury and illness.

You don't want to hike so hard that you get to camp too exhausted to take care of camp chores and deal with an emergency if necessary. Just as you always want to have an extra dry layer of clothes in the event of very cold weather, you want to maintain some reserve of energy throughout your day and throughout the entirety of the trip.

When hiking, do not take too many rest breaks and do not prolong them. If you have to stop every 20 minutes for a rest break, it means you are either hiking too fast or do not have the physical conditioning or both. You will never get anywhere if you stop every few minutes and you will not develop rhythm and momentum. A good rule of thumb is to hike an hour and rest 10 minutes. You may want to extend the time between breaks depending on how you feel. The point is if you can develop a rhythm of steady hiking with short and regular breaks, you will go farther and faster than the person who stops and starts sporadically. The other problem with long breaks is that you grow sluggish if you rest for more than about 15 minutes. In a group, coordinate your rests so that everyone knows when to put their pack on to go and no one ends up standing there with their 60-pound pack while their friends are still looking for the sunscreen.

It's one thing to find a perfect pace for yourself and quite another to find the right pace for the entire group. If you're lucky, and traveling with a few buddies who are perfectly matched physically, the pace of the whole group may fit the pace of all the individuals. But usually there are discrepancies— fast hikers and slower hikers; people who come from sea level and people who have been living at 6,000 feet; those in perfect health and those having a bad day or suffering from sore feet. Ultimately the pace of your group should be determined by the slowest hiker in your party. Before you even begin your trip, you should agree that the gait along the trail will be comfortable for the weakest member in the group. It can be very frustrating for someone in tremendous physical condition to have to slow his or her pace for the ones less conditioned. Keeping up the morale of the weaker hikers while minimizing the frustration of the fleet hikers is a balancing act and a test of leadership. A pace that exhausts the weak members will, in the long run, lead to morale problems and even health problems. You might consider putting the slowest hiker up front so he or she sets the pace for everyone else. If possible, take some weight from the weaker members and redistribute it among the brutes (this should only be done within reason; try not to carry more than 40 percent of your body weight). A person pushed to his or her physical limits and made to feel a burden to the group will be sapped mentally, demoralized, and will certainly travel more slowly than if he or she were encouraged and accommodated.

The strong hiker can be given the task of map reading or even be put in charge of keeping everyone happy on the trail—call it the trail boss. Navigating tasks or leadership responsibilities will distract him or her from having to walk more slowly.

## WALKING TECHNIQUE

When climbing hills with a heavy pack, some people use what's known as the rest step. The rest step, as the name implies, is a technique that gives the muscles of your leg a momentary rest between strides. It's a simple technique but one that nevertheless takes some getting used to. With the rest step, you momentarily straighten and lock the knee of your weight-bearing leg just before you step onto your other foot. By straightening the weight-bearing leg, instead of always being on a bent leg, you briefly rest your weight on your skeletal structure instead of just your leg muscles.

When carrying a heavy pack (30 percent or more of your body weight) some people like to walk almost flat-footed. Without weight on our backs, we naturally roll up onto the ball of our foot with every step. But with the 50-pound pack, the normal stride onto the toe can wear out calf muscles over the course of a few miles and give you sore spots or blisters on your heels. Walking flat-footed puts more of the work on your thigh muscles and less work on your calf muscles, while also taking some of the pressure off the skin of your heel.

I know great travelers who use the rest step and also walk very flat-footed; I also know great travelers who walk up on their toes as if they are carrying no pack at all. Experiment with these two techniques and find a style that suits you best.

## GROUP MANAGEMENT ON THE TRAIL

If you're just hiking with one or two other people, assigning special roles to each person may seem silly. But with groups of four or more, and with groups of people new to each other's company (on a commercial trip or in an institutional setting, for example), you may find that you can travel more efficiently if you assign tasks. On some NOLS courses, instructors and students pick a leader, a navigator, and a sweeper. The leader's job is to maintain the big picture, make judgments about difficult terrain, keep tabs on the condition of individual group members, and delegate subordinate tasks. The leader should not have to map read and navigate on the trail, as it will distract her from keeping track of the rest of the group. The leader should travel in the middle of the group or circulate from front to back as the day progresses so she can stay in touch with the whole party.

The navigator obviously has to travel at the front of the party. His job is to pick the best route to the destination, be it on trails or off trail. It is the navigator's responsibility to study the route in advance and familiarize himself with the terrain ahead so he can keep the group on track. The navigator should travel with map in hand (or in a convenient pocket) so he can consult his map frequently. He should consult with the group when he has doubts about his route or his location on the map but should not be crowded or constantly second-guessed by the rest of the group. The job of navigator can be difficult and he should be given the time and space to think and plan.

The sweeper travels at the end of the group to make sure no one falls behind or gets lost. While it can sometimes happen that the slowest person ends up being the sweeper, as we have discussed above, always having the slowest person at the end can be demoralizing. The assigned sweeper should stay in touch with the leader and advise her if the pace is too fast.

## DEHYDRATION

In the course of a hard day hiking in the sun, I sometimes feel myself getting grouchy and the smallest things—missing a trail junction or tripping over a tree root—irritate me. If my campmates are lucky, I recognize one of the symptoms of dehydration and stop and drink some water. Acutely dehydrated, I can find reason to grumble about nearly anything under the sun.

Perhaps the second most used dictum of NOLS instructors—after "Use your judgment"—is "Drink some water." I have seen fellow instructors recommend a chug from the water bottle for ailments ranging from fatigue to headaches. It's good advice. The water in our bodies carries nutrients, oxygen, enzymes, and hormones, controls body temperature, flushes out toxins, and eliminates waste products. Unless you are in the desert, where water is scarce, staying well hydrated is one of the easiest, cheapest, and most effective things you can do to keep a high level of energy, travel efficiently, and stay healthy.

We constantly lose water from sweating, urinating, breathing, and defecating (human feces are roughly 70 percent water). When we're working hard and sweating heavily we can lose up to a liter of water per hour. At high altitudes where the air is dry, you can dehydrate yourself merely by breathing at rest. If you have ever dried your clothes on a clothesline in the Rocky Mountains, you can imagine that a climate that dries a towel in about twenty minutes can suck you dry pretty fast too.

Under "normal" conditions our bodies' thirst mechanisms—a dry mouth, the hypothalamus, and hormones in the kidneys—stimulate us to drink enough water to stay properly hydrated. But if we are working very hard and sweating profusely, if we are in a very hot or dry climate, or if we have an aggravating condition such as diarrhea, or nausea that causes vomiting, we

> ### Symptoms of Dehydration
>
> ▾ Your urine is dark and you urinate infrequently.
> ▾ You feel dizzy, have a headache, or are nauseated.
> ▾ You have a dry mouth or tongue.
> ▾ You feel thirsty.

have to drink water deliberately and regularly regardless of how thirsty we feel.

Dehydration impairs humans both physically and mentally. As you become dehydrated you lower your blood plasma volume and consequently your heart has to work harder to keep body tissues supplied with blood. The result is a decrease in cardiovascular performance. Dehydrated, your body is also less able to dissipate heat through sweat. Finally, you impair your ability to digest and metabolize food when your body is low on water.

Your physical performance begins to decline when you lose as little as 1 percent of your body's weight in water. If a 150-pound person is down just a quart of water, his body's ability to regulate heat and his exercise performance starts to slip. Down three quarts of water, that 150-pound person will lose 20 to 30 percent of his exercise performance. The following table shows water loss as it relates to performance and symptoms.

Studies have shown that prehydration—drinking extra water before a strenuous activity—will also help performance. Fortunately the best thing to drink—and certainly the simplest and cheapest—is just plain cold water. Studies have shown that the carbohydrate-electrolyte enhanced drinks such as Gatorade and ERG are no more easily absorbed by the intestines than just

*Figure 6-1 Water Loss as a Percentage of Body Weight Related to Performance and Symptoms\**

| | |
|---|---|
| 0% | Normal heat regulation and performance. |
| 1% | Thirst is stimulated, heat regulation during exercise is altered, performance begins to decline. |
| 2%–3% | Further decrease in heat regulation, increased thirst, worsening performance. |
| 4% | Exercise performance cut by 20–30%. |
| 5% | Headache, irritability, "spaced-out" feeling, fatigue. |
| 6% | Weakness, severe loss of thermoregulation. |
| 7% | Collapse is likely unless exercise is stopped. |

\*"Nutrition for Cyclists," Grandjean & Ruud, *Clinics in Sports Medicine*, Vol. 13(1): 235–246, Jan. 1994.

## Tips for Staying Hydrated

▼ Prehydrate: Drink extra water before you start a strenuous activity.

▼ Drink small amounts often.

▼ Drink cool water when possible. Cool water is absorbed more easily by the intestines than warm water is.

▼ Avoid sugary drinks. Sugar impedes the body's ability to absorb fluid.

▼ Make it easy for yourself to drink water often by keeping your water bottle in a convenient place or by using a dromedary bag.

▼ Make drinking water a habit. If you just rely on your sense of thirst, chances are you will get behind in your hydration. Make a point of drinking at least 8 ounces of water for every half hour of strenuous activity.

▼ Avoid alcohol and caffeine. Both are diuretics and cause the body to lose water through urination.

plain water. Some studies even suggest that the extra sugar and electrolytes in these drinks impairs the body's ability to absorb fluid. The one advantage the commercial drinks have is that their sweet, fruity flavors entice some people to drink more than they would if the stuff in their bottle was just plain water.

Alcohol and caffeine inhibit one of the kidney's hormones that regulates water loss, so drinking either alcohol or caffeine will accelerate dehydration.

The table below shows the amount of water you should drink to stay healthy and maintain your energy.

### NUTRITION

According to a study cited in *Exercise Physiology: Energy, Nutrition, and Human Performance,*[*] an individual weighing 160 pounds, carrying a heavy pack uphill, burns about 625 calories per hour. Compare that to a cross-country skier from the same study, who, skiing across level ground, burns only 612 calories per hour. You need to eat plenty of food to keep

*Figure 6-2 Recommended Daily Water Intake According to Weight*

| Body Weight in Pounds | Liters H$_2$O at Rest |
|---|---|
| 100 | 3 |
| 120 | 3.6 |
| 140 | 4.2 |
| 160 | 4.8 |
| 180 | 5.4 |
| 200 | 6 |

*By William D. McArdle, Frank I. Katch, and Victor L. Katch; William and Wilkins, 1996.

your energy levels up while outdoors. Eat a lot for breakfast, snack all day, and then eat a big dinner to stay warm during the night. It is better to eat several small snacks throughout the day than have a big lunch. It is analogous to feeding a fire continually with small amounts of wood instead of tossing all the wood on the fire in one fell swoop.

In our image-conscious culture, some people treat a trip to the backcountry as yet another opportunity to lose weight. I have been with people who try to diet on what is already a strenuous trip. Inevitably they run low on energy during the day, slow the group, and don't pull their weight. Chances are that with the rigorous exercise you get in the backcountry you'll lose weight no matter what you eat. Regardless, it's not fair to the rest of your teammates to let your energy reserves run low for the sake of your waistline. Leave that silliness back in the city.

# LNT Trail Technique

The LNT principles for hiking in the backcountry are the same as the camping principles:

▾ Hike on durable surfaces.
▾ In heavily used areas, concentrate use.
▾ In remote areas, spread use.

The best place to hike whenever you're in the near vicinity is on an established trail. Trails are laid out to get you through the backcountry without creating too much erosion. Land managers have built and maintained trails connecting popular destinations and have contoured the trails to make reasonable walking grades.

Someday when you're walking down the trail in the backwoods, you'll come to a point where the trail forks into two, three, or even four parallel trails that continue for 50 yards or so and then rejoin to form the main trail. What you're seeing is likely the result of hikers walking off the trail to avoid a muddy spot. Depressions along the trail get muddy in the same spots year after year and lots of hikers step off the trail to stay out of the mud. The problem with sidestepping all the mud puddles is that it turns once single-lane trails into multilane freeways much more prone to erosion. While it's human to want to avoid the wet spots, do your best to stay on the trails, even if it means getting your boots muddy. Wearing waterproof boots and a pair of gaiters will make you more likely to stay on the trail regardless of the conditions.

Some hikers leave the trail on steep switchbacks and take shortcuts straight up the hill. The shortcutters make vertical trails of their own that make perfect channels for water runoff and heavy-duty erosion. While you may knock off a few minutes with a shortcut, the switchbacks in the trail were put there to keep the water from running down the mountain in torrents.

If you decide to leave the main trail system on your trip, you have to be more careful how you travel. First of all, instead of walking single file as you would on a trail, it's best to spread out and take separate paths through a pristine meadow or forest. Walking in one line through a pristine area starts the trace of a new trail, which is likely to be followed by the next travelers who come along. Spreading out and walking on durable surfaces will leave scant trace of your crossing and, with luck, the area will recover before a new trail is developed.

If you do decide to travel off trail, find the toughest surfaces you can to walk on. Just as with campsites, certain surfaces are more resistant to foot traffic. Dry meadows, forests with little understory, sedges and grasses, rock, snowfields, and dry creekbeds are the most resistant hiking surfaces. The most delicate surfaces are forests with thick understory, wet meadows, alpine cushion plants, and steep slopes (due to the cutting and tearing action boots make on ascents or descents).

Avoid walking on trace trails or trails just being developed. It's not always clear which is an established trail and which is the work of single-line hikers walking through a pristine area. Use your best judgment.

### Interview with an Outdoor Photographer

Jeff Foott is one of the world's premier wildlife photographers and wildlife cinematographers. His photography has appeared in *National Geographic, Audubon,* and *Smithsonian* magazines. The BBC named Foott wildlife photographer of the year and his cinematography on killer whales was nominated for an Emmy award. Foott lives in Jackson Hole, Wyoming.

In this interview, I asked Jeff to address the novice-to-intermediate photographer.

**Q:** What kind of film do you recommend for the outdoor photographer?

**A:** I recommend 100 ASA slide film such as Fujichrome or Ektachrome E100. It's fine grained and if you need faster speed for the low-light situations, you can "push" it a stop to 200 ASA. If you're going to shoot in the outdoors, you should know how to "push" your film. If you're using 100 ASA film, set the ASA on your camera for 200 and tell the lab to push the film one stop. I have even pushed 100 ASA film two stops to 400 with good results. [Note: you can't usually change the ASA on point-and-shoot cameras.] One of the reasons I recommend slide film is that you can make good prints from slide film but you can't make good slides from print film.

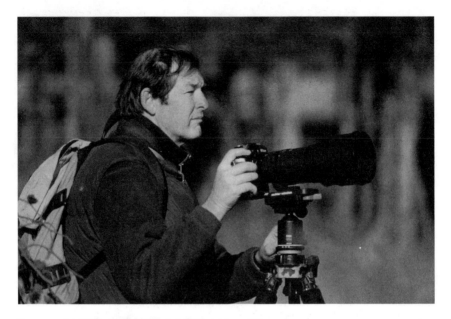

Renowned wildlife photographer Jeff Foott. *Janet Urban*

**Q:** What sort of equipment and lenses do you recommend for the backpacker?

**A:** It's a matter of weight versus quality. If you really want to go light, the new point-and-shoots are pretty damn good. But if you carry an SLR [single lens reflex] camera, you might as well carry a small tripod. I would recommend a wide-angle lens (24mm–28mm) and a 55mm or 60mm macro lens for the close-up shots. If I could only take one telephoto lens, I would go with a 105mm. If you're really going to shoot outdoors a lot, you might consider getting a Nikon FM2. It's really light and works well in cold weather.

I would also recommend taking a polarizing filter. Foliage and the crystals on rock faces give off a lot of glare. The polarizing filter will help cut out the glare and will saturate the colors. It will make the sky darker and bluer. I always use it on mountains, rocks, and vegetation.

**Q:** What advice do you have for shooting in bad weather?

**A:** It's no big deal, really. Cameras these days can handle most anything. If it's really cold, I take some of that flexible Styrofoam packing material and put it on the parts of the equipment that I have to handle when shooting pictures—tripod legs, the focus ring on the lens, and things like that. I cover the Styrofoam with cotton gaffer's tape.

**Q:** What can the budding photographer do to improve his or her composition?

**A:** If you divide your photo into thirds both vertically and horizontally, you get a sort of tic-tac-toe grid with four points of intersection. Those are the strongest compositional points and where you should put your subject in the photo. The center of the grid is the weakest point of composition. The biggest mistake people make

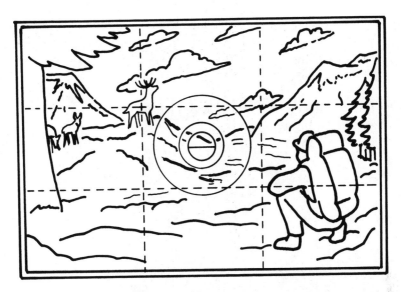

The view through your camera. Don't center all your subjects. Dividing your viewfinder in thirds vertically and horizontally gives an imaginary tic-tac-toe grid and four points of intersection. Try putting your subject on one of those points for stronger composition.

with horizons is to put them right in the middle of the photo. The horizon should go at the top third or bottom third of the photo.

**Q:** What should the photographer know about approaching wildlife?

**A:** Simply this: Don't harass the wildlife. If you disturb the natural wildlife behavior, that, by definition, is harassment.

**Q:** What's your advice on getting the right exposure?

**A:** Getting the correct exposure is an art. One thing I can suggest is to avoid metering off the sky even if the sky will be part of your composition. Meter off neutral colors on the ground in front of you, and then compose your picture with that same meter reading. That usually works pretty well.

## Precarious Terrain and Objective Hazards

Your route may be so easy that the only terrain you cross is rolling hill and lightly perfumed dale, but even if that is the case there are still objective hazards out there. An objective hazard is a danger that exists in nature independent of anything you do. Objective hazards include poor weather, swift rivers, rock fall, and avalanches. You can manage or mitigate objective hazards, but you can't eliminate them. You can't stop a lightning storm, but you can get off the ridge when it comes in. Your job when encountering an objective hazard, be it a snowfield or a raging river, is to first use your judgment and decide if tackling the hazard is within your competence. Then your job is to use the best techniques possible to minimize the danger.

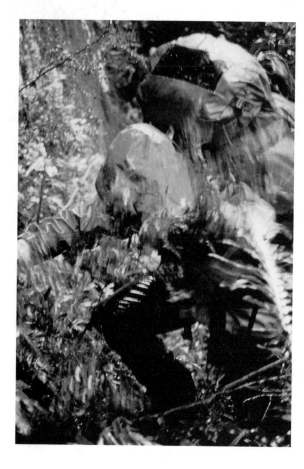

Bushwhacking through the wilds of Chilean Patagonia on a NOLS semester course. *Deborah Sussex*

## RIVER CROSSINGS

On a topographical map, a river is but a thin blue line that tells little about the speed, force, and volume of the water. When you spread your maps out and plan your route, you can estimate a river's size by looking at the amount of terrain it drains, but you won't know for sure until you get to the river itself. River crossings are at once exhilarating, challenging, frustrating, dangerous, and satisfying. On a nice summer day, crossing a river can be the highlight of the trip. On a cold, rainy day when the footing is slick and the current strong, crossing a river can be dangerous and frustrating.

In heavily used areas, land managers sometimes construct foot bridges

## Estimating the Size of a River from Reading Your Map

It's not easy to estimate the size and strength of a river just by looking at your map, but you can infer something of its scale by looking at the river's watershed—the entire system of drainages feeding it. The river that drains several large basins, each of which has perennial streams or rivers, will be bigger than the river that only drains small gullies and intermittent streams.

across rivers, so you can just stroll across. But in wilder areas, you don't have the advantage of a stout bridge; knowing how to evaluate rivers and how to choose whether to cross, where to cross, and how to cross a river safely need to be part of your repertoire as an outdoorsperson. The most important tool to have as a river crosser—even more important than strong legs and a big stick—is judgment and respect for the water. If you can evaluate a river crossing and make a sound decision as to whether or not you should cross it, you will enjoy the mountains longer than the guy with the huge legs, no fear, and no judgment.

Small streams and creeks can be crossed with little trouble, but you have

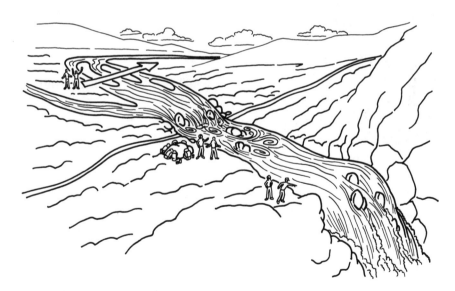

If you have doubts about crossing a river, scout upstream and downstream until you find a place you feel comfortable crossing. You may have to scout a mile or more before you find a good ford. Scout in pairs and have an agreed upon time for returning. Always consider the consequences of the runout—where the river would take you if you fell. Sometimes you can walk upstream, cross a small tributary and then the main channel with less volume.

to be willing to get your feet wet. If there is a dry, sturdy log nearby, or a series of stable rocks that brook the crossing, there's no reason not to take advantage of them. But some people go to great and dangerous lengths to keep their feet dry—crossing slimy logs or making great leaps between moss-covered rocks—and usually end up in the drink anyway. If keeping your boots dry means risking a turned ankle or worse, it's just not worth it. One NOLS instructor I've worked with deliberately walks across every stream of consequence *in* the water just to make the point to his students.

### Scouting

The bigger, faster river crossings are more involved. The first thing to do when you come to a strong river is to scout around for the easiest crossing site. You may find a widening in the river just a quarter mile upstream that poses far less risk than where the trail meets the river. If the river is strong and dangerous, you may need to spend considerable time scouting up and down the river—even a mile or two. Break up your party into two groups: one to scout downstream and the other upstream. Have an arranged time to meet back at the packs.

A rough rule of thumb is that you can only cross rivers that travel at your walking speed or slower. It may give you perspective on the river's speed to throw a stick or pine cone upstream and walk alongside the object as it descends. The speed of a river can be deceiving when the river runs through a smooth stretch.

Listen for the telltale signs of stones or boulders rolling down the riverbed. If you hear a deep rumbling and clinking sound, it means the current is strong enough to sweep large stones downstream. That should give you some idea of the river's strength and that you will have the added risk of rocks hitting you in the shins.

If you have doubts about the strength of the river, take your pack off and test the waters without your pack. Find a large pole and probe the current ahead of you. The pole will also help you probe the depth so you don't accidentally step into a deep hole. You may want to hold the pole in one hand and link hands with a friend to give you support and perhaps drag you back out if the current is too strong.

Once you find a potential crossing, consider where the river would take you if you lost your footing and fell. Your crossing may seem perfectly safe but if it is perched above big rapids, then you need to find another crossing. Potential hazards downstream of your crossing include rapids, strainers (trees that have fallen into the river), cataracts, and steep banks that would prevent you from climbing out of the water.

Once you do decide to cross the river, waterproof the essential items in your pack such as your sleeping bag, food, camera, and warm clothes. Take your socks off, but leave your boots on to give you the support you need.

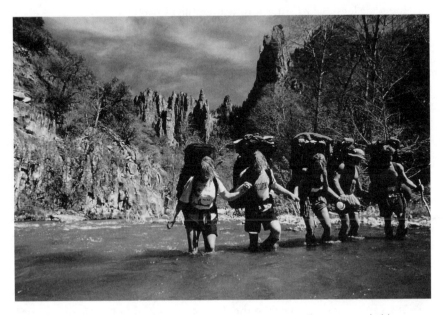

A good way to cross a river with a slow to moderate current is in a group holding hands. This group of NOLS students is crossing the Gila River in Arizona's Gila Wilderness. *John McConnell*

### Crossing Methods

There are several methods for crossing rivers. The method you choose will depend on the strength of the river and the strength of the individuals in the group. But whether you are crossing alone or in a group, the following tips will help you stay balanced and focused.

- ▾ When crossing a river, face upstream into the current. Facing upstream puts you in a stronger, more balanced position, forces the weight onto the balls of your feet, and allows you to watch for dangerous objects floating downstream.
- ▾ Don't stare at the current straight in front of you. Flowing water can be hypnotic or cause a sort of vertigo. Shift your gaze from point to point, keeping an eye on your destination, the water upstream (for obstacles), and the footing below you for holes or irregularities in the bed.
- ▾ Wear your boots. Not only will your boots give you better footing, they

will also protect you against rolling rocks being carried downstream by the current.

▾ Do not cross one leg behind or in front of the other as you traverse the river. Instead, shuffle your feet like a tennis or basketball player. Crossing your legs makes you more vulnerable to tripping.

▾ Hipbelts: When and whether to use the hipbelt on your pack while crossing a river is a contentious subject. The advantage of using your hipbelt while crossing a river is that it stabilizes your pack by keeping the weight from shifting so much, and thereby helps you stay balanced. The disadvantage is that if you fall while crossing you may not be able to get your pack off to save yourself. You can well imagine the danger of having a 40-, 50-, or 60-pound pack tightly strapped to your body while you're trying to escape a strong river current. Here are some rules of thumb for using a hipbelt. If the water is above your knees, take your hipbelt off before crossing; or if the current is strong enough that you decide to cross in a group, then take your hipbelt off.

▾ Shoulder straps: Even with your hipbelt off, it can be very difficult to shed your pack. Slightly loosening your shoulder straps makes it easier to get your pack off in an emergency.

▾ Using a stick: A strong stick can be your best friend when crossing a river. You can use a stick to probe the depths in front of you and you can use the stick for balance. Find a stick from five to seven feet long, and make sure it is truly strong (i.e., no rotten sections or cracks). Some people use collapsible ski poles or walking sticks to help them cross rivers. Collapsible poles are fine for moderate rivers but should be used with caution on strong rivers simply because they tend to do just what their name suggests: collapse.

The advantage of crossing a river alone is that if you get swept off your feet, you won't drag your teammates with you. The corollary is of course that your teammates can't catch you either. Crossing the river alone makes sense in slow currents when everyone in the group is reasonably strong and balanced.

In stronger currents, consider crossing the river in a small group of two to five people. The simplest way is to link arms or hold hands. The strongest person should go first as he or she will have the best chance of recovering and turning back if the river is too strong. If you cross in a group of three, put the weakest person in the middle so the stronger members on the outside can support him.

You can also cross rivers in a single line, a technique also known as the "eddy method." This style may be your best choice in the really strong rivers. Put your strongest members at the front and the back of the line. The advantage here is that those in the middle are buffered from the current. The person in the front of the line should have a large stick to lean on. The next person in line, number two, puts his hand on the shoulders or pack of person number one both to support him and to put pressure on that person's feet, should he or she have trouble with the footing. The third person stands di-

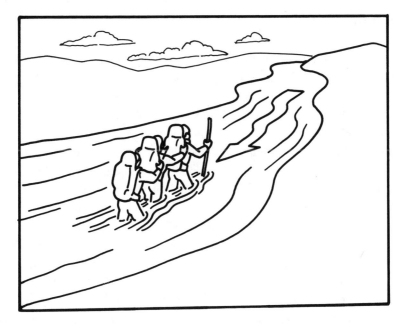

Eddy-method river crossing. In strong currents, joining the team together in a sort of human train can make the going easier. Put a strong person at the head of the chain with a stick to lean on, if possible. Each person helps the member in front of him by grasping the pack and offering firm support. The group moves in tandem.

rectly behind the second person, also with his hands on the pack or shoulders in front. The entire line moves across the river in tandem like a centipede.

### When and Where

If you are doing your trip in the western United States, remember that the river will be strongest in the afternoon after the sun has melted the snow up in the high country. You might have better luck crossing the river in the early morning before the sun hits. The water can be ice cold but also lower and slower. The time of year affects the river's flow as well. In mountainous parts of the world, the spring usually brings the fastest waters as the snow melts.

Rivers get smaller the higher you hike up the valley because they have fewer and fewer tributaries. If the spot where you want to cross looks too big, take a look at your map and see if there is a tributary joining the river nearby. Perhaps you can hike up to that tributary, cross it, and then cross the main river.

Look for braids in the river where the total volume of water is divided into two or three channels.

### In the Event of a Fall

If you do fall and are swept downstream, you need to be able to ditch your pack and swim for shore. Try to get your feet downstream. You can use your feet to ward off rocks and your hands to paddle toward shore or away from hazards.

To people, such as kayakers, who habituate the waters, perhaps the most dangerous hazard is the strainer. Should you find yourself heading toward a strainer without the possibility of avoiding it, your goal is to avoid getting sucked under it. River guides advise actually swimming toward the strainer to pick up speed so you can better swim up onto it.

The first in your group to cross the river can act as spotters downstream from the crossing. They should be prepared to help fallen members escape the current but should keep in mind their own limits in wading out to help. If you can't reach the downed person with just your arm, try a stick or a pile jacket. If you are a spotter on the side of a river and need to rescue someone in the water, there is a good mantra to remember: "Reach, throw, then row or go." It is safest to rescue a person in the water by extending a stick or even a jacket if they are close enough. Failing that, throw them a rope if you can. And finally, only as a last resort should you swim to their assistance.

River crossings are one of the more dangerous parts of your travel day. Always be ready to change your route or turn back if the river is too strong.

## CROSSING BOULDERS, TALUS, AND SCREE

Crossing a boulder field, you need to be in balance and ready to react to a wobbly rock. If you know you have a long boulder field to cross, you may want to rest, eat, and drink before crossing it. Tuck in loose clothing or straps that might trip you. If the boulders are very large—say six feet tall and over—you may need free hands to help you negotiate the terrain. If you're carrying a walking stick, you may want to put it in your pack to free your hands. Picking a line through a boulder field is akin to picking a line down a mogul field (if you're a skier). Look ahead often and try to pick out your line two or three

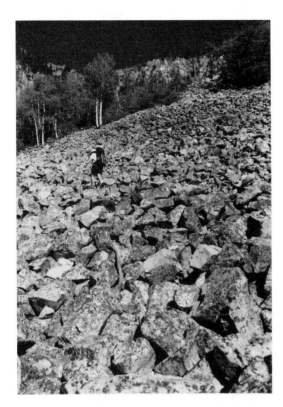

Picking a line through a boulder field is akin to picking a line down a mogul field on a ski slope. You may want to rest, snack, and hydrate yourself before crossing a difficult boulder field so that your concentration is at its best. *Mark Harvey*

steps ahead of the game. Step near the center of rocks; stepping on the edges may flip an unstable boulder.

## ROCKFALL

If you have ever heard the menacing whir and hum of a free-falling rock, you know the deadly speed and force of rockfall. Falling rocks are one of the leading causes of accidents in mountaineering. Probably the only way to completely eliminate the danger of rockfall is to stay out of the mountains. But you can reduce the danger by knowing something about the nature of falling rocks—the where and when—and then by choosing your route and timing carefully.

Any route that is steep and rocky at least has the potential of falling rocks. But some steep and rocky areas are much less stable than others. You can begin your evaluation of the route by looking for clues of recent action. Recall the saying "rolling stones gather no moss." If you see piles of rubble and fresh scars at the base of steep pitches, you have obvious evidence that the area is prone to rockfall. Rock piles covered with moss and lichen, by contrast, suggest more stability.

Look at the rock itself. Igneous rocks such as granite and andesite are more stable than metamorphic rock such as schist, slate, and gneiss, and sedimentary rocks such as shale and sandstone. You don't have to identify the rocks by their taxonomy to determine their strength. Touch the rock and look at it. Can you peel chunks of it off the walls around you, or is it strong enough to chin yourself on?

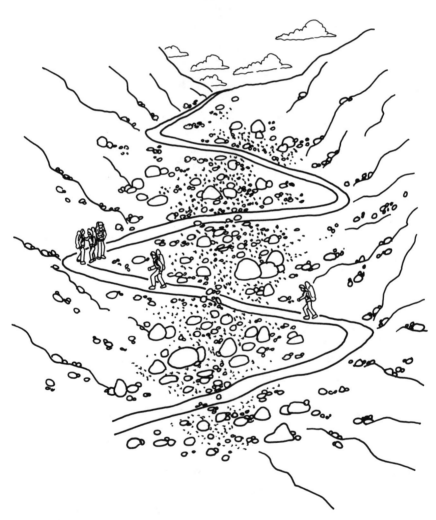

On steep switchbacks with the possibility of rockfall, "corral" your group on the corners so that you don't have one hiker kicking rocks on hikers below.

Climate, weather, season, and time of day affect the stability of rocks too. Areas that receive lots of freezing and thawing will be less stable than moderate climates with the same rock composition. Spring thaws dislodge rocks that have been kept stable by winter's ice. The daily cycle of freezing and thawing affects rockfall too. The slopes are most stable in the early morning before sun begins melting snow and ice. East slopes receive the first sun and thus the rock will begin to loosen on those slopes first. South slopes follow and finally west slopes.

You can allay the danger of falling rock in several ways:

- Try to stay on ridges and avoid couloirs. Rocks, like water, follow couloirs.
- Plan your route so that you are crossing the areas prone to falling rock during the early morning before the ice has melted.
- Do not take breaks in the middle of the combat zone. Find a sheltered place to take a break.
- Keep your group close together so falling rocks don't have a chance to gain speed. On switchbacks you greatly reduce the risks of rockfall by keeping everyone on the same zig or the same zag and then "corralling" the group at the turns. In other words, every time the trail makes its switchback, wait for the entire group to catch up before taking the turn. It takes longer to travel this way, but you ensure that no one is below you.
- If you have to cross an area with rockfall potential, take the shortest route across that exposed area even if it means making the other part of your route longer.
- If you have a helmet, wear it across the area in doubt.
- If you see a rockfall and it has the potential to hit anyone in the group, yell "Rock!" loudly. Better to cast the false alarm than to study the weight and speed of the missile as it gains terminal velocity. At that point the person below will have only milliseconds to react.
- Make sure members of the group know what to do when a rock falls in their direction. If you're at the base of a cliff or near a big boulder, press up close to the steepest part. Rocks falling down steep slopes or cliffs tend to get bounced away from the slope. If you're not near a cliff, try to hide behind the nearest big tree or large boulder.
- Tread lightly. Big packs, big boots, and fatigue make clumsy feet. Clumsy feet kick rocks. Concentrate on your foot placement when there is a dangerous rock field.

## SNOW

Crossing snowfields high in the mountains is one of the great joys of back-packing and mountaineering. The moment of finding a snowfield in the middle of July, when all about you is hot and dry, can make the whole trip worthwhile. But snow is a plastic form, hard to judge at its best and downright deadly at its worst. Climbers speak of "antiseptic granite," a form of rock that is stable, predictable, and strong. Snow is the antiseptic granite's opposite: more mysterious and harder to judge. A thorough discussion of avalanches, use of crampons, and ice climbing is beyond the scope of this book, but every hiker should know something about snow in its myriad forms and be alert to the hazards of crossing snow and ice.

### Postholing

Postholing means plunging up to your crotch when the snow surface you're crossing gives way. Typically you'll posthole on spring or summer days when the sun has had time to melt the surface. Postholing is frustrating and even dangerous if you are not expecting it. The danger is in breaking through the crust with a fully loaded pack and landing on a straightened leg. The weight of the pack and the sudden impact on the leg can hyperextend a knee or sprain an ankle. If you cross a snowfield, be aware that you may break through and posthole; you'll have a better chance of landing with a bent knee and softening your fall. If you suspect a weak crust and the possibility of postholing, don't put all your weight on your foot at once; gradually weight your foot and test the surface. When crossing a snowfield watch for tips of boulders and bushes. The snow often forms cavities around plants and rocks that make perfect spots to posthole. The edges of snowfields are typically less firm (from melting) than the center, so be ready for the crust to break both when first stepping onto the snowfield and when exiting the snowfield. Snowfields are firmest in the early morning before the sun has had a chance to melt the surface.

### Self-Arrest on Snow

Slips and slides on snow are another leading cause of accidents, injuries, and fatalities in the mountains. A snowfield with a 30-degree pitch at the top and a 5-degree runout may be a perfectly safe place to cross and even glissade. But a snowfield with a 30-degree pitch that sits above a boulder field or a cliff may be completely unsafe for those traveling without ice axes and good self-arresting skills. The runout, all the terrain below the snowfield, determines in large part whether or not you should cross it. Look for boulders, drops, and

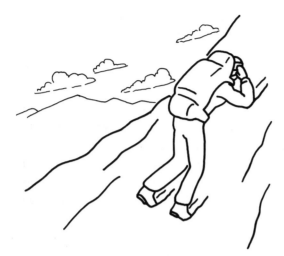

Self-arrest without an ice axe. The time it takes you to arrest depends on snow hardness, the pitch of the slope, the weight of your pack, and your technique. Arresting on a hard, steep slope requires an ice axe.

trees that sit in the path you would take if you were to fall. The firmness of the snow also determines whether or not you'll be able to self-arrest. Early in the morning, after a cold night, snowfields can be rock hard. It is very difficult to slow a fall on frozen snow. Test the conditions with a few kicks of your boot before crossing a field.

If you plan to do a lot of traveling on glaciers or snowfields, you need to learn to stop yourself in the event of a slip or stumble—self-arresting. To really self-arrest quickly on a steep slope requires an ice axe and lots of practice. But you can self-arrest on moderate grades without an axe and the skill for doing so is a good one to know and practice. On some NOLS courses we find a snowfield with a safe runout and spend several hours practicing crossing techniques and self-arrests. Students practice self-arresting with and without an axe from all positions of a fall—on their backs, on their stomachs, head downhill, and feet downhill. It takes practice on real snow to learn to stop yourself, but it's good fun learning and the skill may one day save you from injury or death.

To arrest without an axe you need to somehow get onto your stomach with your feet downhill and dig your elbows and your toes into the snow. It is very difficult to arrest if your whole body is flat against the snow. To stop effectively you need to get the most force onto your elbows and toes, by raising your seat up into the air away from the snow and creating a sort of bent bridge between your feet and your elbows. Spreading your feet slightly wider than hip width will give you more stability as you arrest.

You may get lucky and fall right onto your stomach with your feet downhill. But you might also stumble and fall onto your back with your head downhill. No matter how you fall, you have to right yourself to the correct position.

### Walking on Snow

On moderately pitched snowfields, you can walk flat-footed and still get enough traction to ascend or cross a slope. Often the most comfortable style for ascending snowfields is a duck-footed walk. But as the snow gets steeper, you need to kick steps with the toe of your boot (unless you are wearing crampons). The most energy-efficient way to kick steps is to swing the whole leg back in an exaggerated motion and then swing it forward into the snow, letting the weight and momentum of your boot break the snow. You shouldn't have to kick a huge platform with each step, just a small ledge to step up onto. The leader's steps should be nearly level ledges that the person behind can step up onto without having to contort the ankle up or down. The leader's strides should also be small enough to be comfortable for the smaller hikers in the group.

There's no sense having everyone in the party waste energy by kicking their own new steps. The leader can kick the steps, while the people in the back follow along, being careful to improve the steps with their own boots. Because leading up snowfields is strenuous, the lead position should be changed as often as is necessary. If the snow is so hard that you can't kick a step with one swing of your leg, you should not be crossing the slope without crampons and an ice axe.

You can descend moderate snowfields glissading, which means sliding down on your feet as if you're skiing on your boots. But once again, pay careful attention to the pitch of the slope and the runout. If you're in doubt, play it conservatively and find an alternate route or plunge step down the snow.

Plunge stepping is akin to the goose stepping of Prussian armies. Facing downhill, you swing your leg out in front of you, straighten it, and then violently plunge your heel through the crust. The best position for plunge stepping is to be slightly bent over at the waist—nose over toes.

### Avalanches

When I was in my late teens, an avalanche nearly buried me while I was backcountry skiing with my brother and a friend. We went skiing on a very steep gully that we had skied for years without problems. I went first and skied about 400 feet down the powder and then stopped to watch my brother

## Avalanche Danger

▼ Heavy snowfall: Snowfall of an inch or more per hour or over a foot of snow in a 24-hour period. Eighty percent of avalanches happen during or shortly after a heavy snowfall.
▼ Slopes with an incline between 25 and 55 degrees. Slopes between 30 and 45 degrees are especially susceptible to slides.
▼ Treeless couloirs and bowls.
▼ Slopes with a point of convexity.
▼ North-facing slopes in the winter. South-facing slopes in the spring (Northern Hemisphere).

and friend. Looking up the hill, I saw a puff of white below where they were standing and knew immediately an avalanche had started. Nearly without thinking, I turned my skis downhill, got some speed, and skied up and out of the gully just as the avalanche blew by me. The speed and power of this avalanche stunned me. It covered the 400 feet in just a few seconds, had chunks in it the size of a sofa, and flattened every small tree in its path. If the thing had caught me I assume I wouldn't be here today writing about it.

In retrospect, we had no business skiing there that day. It had snowed heavily that week and the terrain had every characteristic of wanting to slide: It was a steep gully, had no trees and was snow-laden. Having skied the chute so many times over the years, we had become blasé about the dangers and we couldn't resist the powder.

This is not a book on technical mountaineering so my discussion of avalanches here will be brief. But even if you're just a summer hiker, it's worth knowing the basics of avalanches.

Avalanches are most common on slopes with a pitch of between 30 and 45 degrees, though they frequently occur on pitches ranging from 25 to 55 degrees. Slopes shallower than 25 degrees rarely slide simply because they lack the grade. Slopes steeper than 55 degrees don't normally collect enough snow to make them avalanche prone.

There are two types of avalanches: slab avalanches and loose-snow avalanches. When the snow is cohesive enough to slide as a single unit, you can have a slab avalanche. Heavy new snow and wind-deposited snow often form a dense slab that will break off and slide given the right conditions. Loose-snow avalanches form from snow that does not have the structural integrity of the slab. They start at one point and develop speed and volume as they descend.

Slab avalanches are likely to occur when the outermost layer sits on a weak or slippery layer below it. The weak layer can be a grassy hillside, a layer of ice, a wind or sun crust, or hoar crystals formed during cold nights. The hoar crystals make a weak layer because they bond poorly with the adjoining layers and shear easily as well.

Avalanches are most likely to start on treeless slopes, couloirs, and bowls. Convex slopes are particularly prone to slides because the shape creates a point of tension in the snow layers. In the Northern Hemisphere, north-facing slopes are more apt to slide in the winter and south-facing slopes are more apt to slide in the spring. In the winter, the north-facing slopes are colder and develop more hoar frost. What's more, the cold temperatures mean that the north-facing snow takes longer to consolidate and stabilize. But in the spring, the south-facing slopes are made unstable by the meltwater.

The information here is a cursory introduction to avalanches and is meant only to help you identify the hazards should you be traveling on snow-covered mountains in the spring. Even the most experienced winter mountaineers can't predict avalanches with certainty. If you plan to do any winter mountaineering, you would do well to study the subject in depth with books and classes.

## Subjective Hazards

In a recent conversation I had with Drew Leemon, director of risk management at NOLS, he said he considered subjective hazards—the human factor—to be just as dangerous as objective hazards, such as rivers, avalanches, or rockfall, in backcountry travel. As the name suggests, subjective hazards have everything to do with human judgment and human error. If a person attempts a peak despite deteriorating weather and suffers hypothermia, was it the objective hazard of the storm or the subjective hazard of the person's decision to push ahead that caused the injury? As Phil Powers points out in his book *NOLS Wilderness Mountaineering,* "It should be clear that it is impossible to separate objective from subjective dangers completely."*

A person's frame of mind, judgment, and experience all determine the level of subjective hazard. Someone who pays thousands of dollars and devotes a lot of time to attempt a mountain summit may suspend good judgment and take unnecessary risks in trying for the summit despite dangerous weather conditions or personal limitations.

Fatigue, hunger, and dehydration all add to the subjective hazards of backcountry travel. The exhausted and poorly nourished person simply can't make the same good decisions she would make if she were well rested and

*Phil Powers, *NOLS Wilderness Mountaineering,* Stackpole Books, 1993, p. 46.

well fed. Tired campers aren't usually as vigilant in doing the camp chores: pitching a taut tent, dressing well to stay warm, staying abreast of the navigation, etc.

A group's ability to work well together and communicate effectively plays a role as well. The group that discusses problems, plans, and the environmental factors will likely make better decisions than individuals would. When communication breaks down, sometimes egos get in the way of clear thinking and clear planning. Likewise, the competence of the group's leader makes a huge difference in determining the hazards of travel. Inexperienced travelers following a leader with poor judgment put themselves at risk regardless of the objective hazards.

Sometimes subjective hazards manifest themselves in the early planning of the trip. The food, equipment, and maps you bring, along with your contingency plans, may determine whether or not your party members stay safe and healthy. Bringing bad gear or not having a contingency plan is human error, not something wrought by nature.

The objective hazards of the backcountry will always be there, be it a weather system or a steep rock face. But our state of mind, our judgment, our skill level, and our planning all help determine just how safe or dangerous the trip is.

## Trail Etiquette

When you travel in a large group, it's especially important that you be considerate of your fellow hikers. In fact, the first thing to do when traveling in a large group is to break up into smaller groups. There is something disheartening about encountering a group of ten hikers out on the trail. Somehow, meeting two groups of five is less offensive.

Take your lunch breaks and rest breaks well off the trail. No one likes to have to trip through someone's salami and cheese.

Usually the group going uphill has the right of way over the group going downhill. But if you're young and strong, you probably have the agility to cede the way to everyone coming your way.

## Meeting Horsepackers

If you are traveling on foot and meet horsepackers on the trail, keep it in mind that you have more mobility than those on the horses. Therefore, you should cede the trail to those traveling with stock. Most horses in the mountains have had enough experience to take backpackers in stride, but certain horses spook when confronted with hikers. On hills, step to the downside of the trail so if the horse does spook it will run up the hill instead of down the hill, giving the rider a better chance of bringing the horse back into control.

# Smoking and Alcohol

When it comes right down to it, wilderness areas are one of the last public domains where you can light up without being told by a firm voice that smoking is not allowed. If you take a NOLS course, you have to leave the smokes and the booze behind (for a variety of reasons), but for some people—in the words of Willie Nelson—"The reasons to quit don't outnumber all the reasons why." The fact is, many people choose to bring tobacco and alcohol on their trips and do so responsibly. All we can advise you of are the peculiar hazards associated with drugs, alcohol, and smoking in the wilderness and of some precautions to take.

Carelessly flick an ash onto the ground in a dry forest and suddenly Marlboro country becomes Yellowstone—the sequel. Take the same precautions with your cigarettes as you would with your campfire. Cast-off cigarette butts give the woods the ambiance of an ashtray or a cigar bar. If you don't want to put the butt in your pocket because of loose tobacco, you can "field strip" it. Take the extinguished butt and roll it vigorously between your fingers so the tobacco is dispersed and all you're left with is the filter. The tobacco will compost nicely and you're left only with a neat filter to pack out in your pocket or your pack.

If you take alcohol with you, at least stay sober when you have dangerous tasks in front of you. Alcohol is a vasodilator and can lead to hypothermia. It gives you a sense of being warm as it dilates blood vessels in your extremities when in fact you are losing heat from your core. What's more, alcohol impairs your most important safety device: your brain. Drinking responsibly in the backcountry, then, means taking the normal precautions you need to take drinking anywhere plus the added precautions you should take in your remote setting.

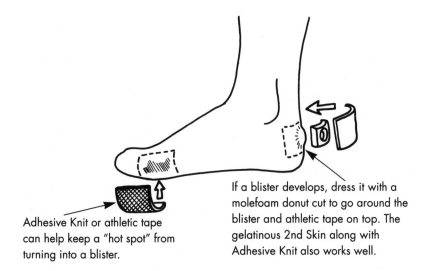

Adhesive Knit or athletic tape can help keep a "hot spot" from turning into a blister.

If a blister develops, dress it with a molefoam donut cut to go around the blister and athletic tape on top. The gelatinous 2nd Skin along with Adhesive Knit also works well.

The best advice with regard to foot care is to stop and take care of "hot spots" before they develop into blisters.

# Foot Care

A blister is your body's way of telling you your boots don't fit, they aren't broken in, or your feet are still too tender for the miles you're covering. The body is kind enough to warn you first with "hot spots," and it's a warning you would do well to heed. The best advice on blisters is to avoid getting them in the first place. The pains you take to care for your feet early on will reward you in doubloons later down the trail. It's especially important that you stop and take care of your feet early in the trip when your feet are still tender. If you take your boots and socks off at rest breaks, you get a chance to look for red areas, which may indicate incipient hot spots. What's more, it allows your feet to cool.

### TREATING BLISTERS

Any time you begin to get a blister, try to figure out a way to relieve pressure on the area. That may mean loosening your boots, removing a pair of socks, or even cutting a hole in your socks around the offending area. If you discover a blister early on when it's still just a hot spot, you can just put a piece of athletic tape or Adhesive Knit (a brand-name adhesive material made of woven fiber that stretches and conforms to the body and is also breathable) over the sore area and usually that will be sufficient protection.

If you wait until the blister develops into a full bubble, the solution becomes more complicated and involves more stuff out of your first-aid kit. Now you really need to relieve the pressure around the sore area. Tod Shimelpfenig, coauthor of *NOLS Wilderness First Aid,* suggests the rule of nickels for deciding whether or not to lance a blister. If the blister is smaller than a nickel, don't lance it because you'll increase the chance of infection. If the blister is bigger than a nickel, it will likely break anyway, so you are better off draining it yourself. Drain the big blisters with a sterilized knife or needle (making a small hole), and then clean them with an antiseptic like zephiran. Cut a piece of molefoam of a size that generously covers the blister. Then cut a smaller hole in the molefoam, making a little donut shape. The donut should fit around the blister, the idea being that the molefoam relieves the pressure from the injury. Fill the molefoam donut with an antibiotic cream and cover the whole donut with athletic tape.

The other solution is to use 2nd Skin directly over the blister, followed by a layer of Adhesive Knit to keep the 2nd Skin in place. 2nd Skin, which can be bought in most drugstores, is a padding that has a high water content. It can be cut into different sizes and shapes and has a slimy, lubricating quality that does a nice job of protecting a sore spot.

You can also do a hybrid of these methods. Cut a molefoam donut, put it around the blister, then cut a piece of 2nd Skin and put it in the donut's hole over the blister. Cover the whole thing with athletic tape.

CHAPTER 7

# Leadership and Expedition Behavior

## Expedition Behavior

In this book we spend several chapters talking about equipment, clothing, camping technique, and travel technique. For good reason: They play an important role in your trip. But human relations play an equally important role. To be blunt, how well you get along with your travelmates can mean the difference between enjoying the wilds or detesting every second of it; between summiting a peak or getting hopelessly lost in the process. That you need to get along and communicate effectively with your travel companions probably seems obvious. We're not talking here about liking each other, but simply getting along and working cooperatively. In the parallel world you might do fine dealing with your colleagues, family, and friends. Perhaps you negotiate labor contracts and can soothe angry unions and high management with tact. Maybe you're a parent and have spent years appeasing your dictatorial toddler, flattering your spouse, and tolerating in-laws. All that speaks well for your people skills, but up in the mountains the entire equation can change. This is not to say the outdoors necessarily aggravates human relations. On the contrary, the sweet air, stunning views, and wildlife sightings often bring out the best in people. Plenty of folks act like angels when in the outback only to metamorphose into antisocial curmudgeons upon returning to town. But traveling in remote areas can try the best of us. Bad weather, fatigue, equipment problems, and getting lost can turn people into monsters.

Outdoor trips force people to live in close quarters for extended periods of time. On a backpacking or a mountaineering trip, you can't just go home at the end of the day and relax in the confines of your own house. At the end of a day on an outdoor expedition, you still have to work as a team setting up camp, making dinner, and keeping the tent in good shape. Nearly every aspect of camping is communal, from the sharing of food to the battle for room in a small tent. At its best, this shared living brings people together in a spirit of camaraderie seldom found in their normal lives. At its worst, the demands of outdoor living can bring people to blows.

There are lots of words and terms to describe the human interactions on an outdoor expedition: process skills, soft skills, people skills, etc. Paul Petzoldt coined the term "expedition behavior" to describe it. After years of mountaineering experience, training soldiers and outdoor leaders, and completing major alpine expeditions, Petzoldt concluded that good or bad expedition behavior often determined a group's destiny even more than technical skills and physical strength. Expeditions with moderate talent but good expedition behavior can achieve greater things than bilious expeditions with all the talent in the world.

Perhaps the first tenet of good expedition behavior is that individuals' basic needs must be met before they can be expected to function at a high level and work well with the group. The most basic human needs are food, water, shelter, and a feeling of security. In other words, be sure that what might seem an attitude problem with one of your teammates isn't just a matter of fatigue, dehydration, hunger, or fear.

The salient needs of human beings are not easy to provide for up in the mountains or out in the desert. Rigorous travel can dehydrate people; a too relaxed attitude toward nutrition can leave people hungry; bad weather combined with poor equipment or poor clothing can make people feel threatened—and for good reason. Poor expedition behavior—sulky, sullen, or stubborn attitudes—may simply be the result of a person not having his salient needs met.

At home, armed with a refrigerator full of food, a hot shower, and a warm bed, taking care of basic needs is much easier. But on outdoor expeditions you would be wise to take on the task seriously. It all begins, of course, with your expedition planning and the wisdom to bring the right rations and sound equipment.

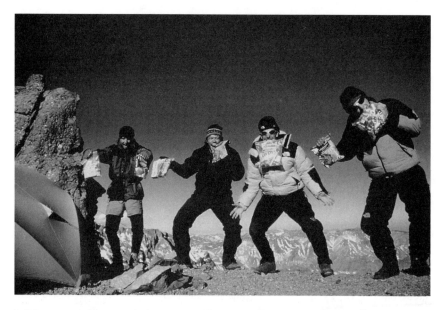

Polish route on Argentina's Aconcagua. Keeping your group working well as a team begins with meeting the salient needs of adequate food and water. Imagine trying to control this bunch without feeding them first. *Pete McBride*

Sometimes when the entire group is tired, hungry, and dehydrated, simple decisions or camp chores take on a certain volatility. At the end of long days, be on guard for your own and others' irritability and take countermeasures to prevent reaching that point by eating and drinking all day. The solution can be as simple as having a snack or a bottle of water.

On a recent bike trip in western Colorado's desert, I noticed that the only real problems we had among the group came at the end of a hot day's riding when people got dehydrated. Low on water, normally reasonable friends sometimes squabbled over nonissues. But this same group immediately settled into good teamwork once its members had chugged a few liters of water. The water seemed to douse the hotheads on any particular day.

After the basic needs of the human organism are met, good expedition behavior springs from all the most decent of human traits: respectfulness, flexibility, tolerance of others, courtesy, politeness, direct communication, self-awareness, open-heartedness, teamwork, sharing, and selflessness. That's quite a laundry list of traits, but what they describe is really just simple decency along with thoughtfulness.

Living and working with others is one of the delights of the outdoors, but the very word "other" reminds us that being thrown into the mix with several people whom we may or may not know well requires a real tolerance of differences, quirks, and even weaknesses. In the argot of today's psychology, a better term might be "mutual adaptation." The term describes a mind-set of not just suffering one another's differences but of respecting, enjoying, and learning from differences. On long expeditions mere tolerance may wear thin and make for brittle relationships and a frosty atmosphere. Fully adapting to other party members and their ways is what gives a group cohesion.

Expedition behavior requires flexibility because the outdoors always has a surprise or two waiting. If you're rigidly set on scaling a peak and seeing its summit, what happens if a teammate is injured, the clouds roll in with a violent storm, or the rest of the group is too exhausted to make the peak? Without flexibility, you may charge ahead despite the weather or despite the fact that you're alone. People intent on achieving their agenda no matter the environmental conditions or the condition of the group can alienate the rest of the team. At worst, the inflexible person can put himself and the others in harm's way with his dogged approach.

Courtesy and politeness smooth the edges of group dynamics. The opportunity to practice courtesy on an expedition can be found at every turn in the trail and at every camp. The courtesies can be as basic as practicing good hygiene, washing your hands before you cook dinner, not strewing your gear all over the tent, and helping someone over a log in the trail. Those are basic courtesies that every person on an expedition should practice. Bringing your friend coffee in the morning, stuffing his sleeping bag, treating a bottle of water—all these acts are nice touches that bring up group morale and, more often than not, are paid back with interest.

Self-awareness gives us the necessary information to change bad habits and to reinforce good ones. Self-awareness comes from reflection and the humility to admit and change your imperfections. An old saying goes, if ten people say you're drunk, you'd better sit down. If your habits and behavior have the same aggravating effect on all of your campmates, you likely need to reflect and make changes.

Recall the interview with John Roskelley earlier in this book: When asked what he attributed his success on major expeditions to, he replied, "My partners." The concept of team and teamwork on outdoor expeditions should be reinforced here. We don't do it alone out there unless we're traveling solo. In the backcountry, a group of disparate personalities, bodies of different sizes and shapes, varying hopes, fears, and expectations, join up to form an organism called the group or the team. The individual never completely loses his singular qualities—and shouldn't—but he does have to adapt his behavior for

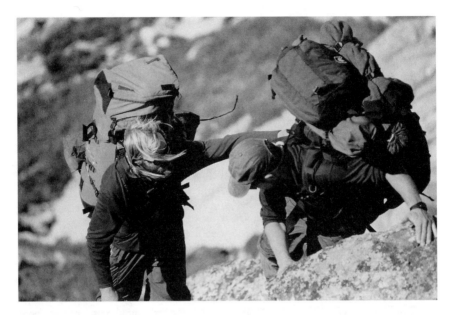

Students on a NOLS course in the Wind River Mountains of Wyoming help each other cross a difficult stretch of terrain. The most successful trips share one common trait: good expedition behavior. *Deborah Sussex*

the good of the group, and his thinking should go from "Is this best for me?" to "Is this best for us?" Putting others first and acting selflessly—it may sound like the stuff of Sunday school, but this all has more to do with practicality than morality. As Paul Petzoldt has said:

> Simply, poor expedition behavior is a breakdown in human relations caused by selfishness, rationalization, ignorance of personal faults, dodging blame or responsibility, physical weakness, and, in extreme cases, not being able to risk one's own survival to insure that of a companion.*

The success, health, and morale of the team matter so much on expeditions that putting the group before your own needs and acting selflessly is a way to ensure the success of the trip.

*Paul Petzoldt, *The New Wilderness Handbook,* W.W. Norton & Company, 1984, p. 168.

### Interview with Molly Doran

In 1991 NOLS honored Molly Doran with the "Outstanding Instructor Award" for years of excellent instruction and directing at the school. Doran has taught more than 250 weeks in the field for NOLS on courses in Kenya, Chile, Alaska, Canada, Wyoming, and Washington State. Presently she is the director of the Leadership Project at NOLS. She earned a master's degree in management and consulting from the Leadership Institute of Seattle.

**Q:** What makes the outdoors a good place to learn leadership?

**A:** In the outdoors, the lessons and consequences of your actions are often immediate. The outdoors reduces your world to a microcosm where there are fewer outside influences to muddy the situation. The lessons are very clear and clean, which is the ideal situation for someone new to being in a leadership role. And people can bite off something manageable and build on that. A person who leads his or her group over some rough terrain on a hiking trip, say, gains confidence and skills that they can use another day in more complex situations.

Compare that to the typical leadership experience a person gets in the city—starting a business, for instance. Running a business, you don't necessarily get direct and immediate feedback. You don't necessarily have a supportive peer group or a mentor. But in the outdoors, the fact that you're living together and dealing with problems that affect the whole group makes the teamwork come more naturally. That's a nice atmosphere for someone to learn leadership. More times than not, it's fun too.

**Q:** Should the typical group of friends going out on a camping trip choose a leader?

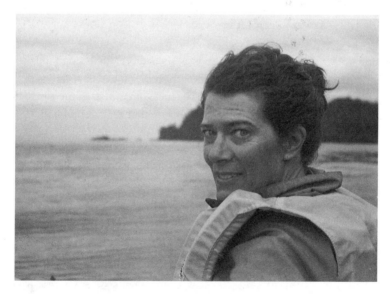

Molly Doran is the director of the Leadership Project at NOLS. *Chris Gerow*

**A:** I think choosing and having a leader makes things so much easier. In my experience, having a leader is less stressful than having everyone guess about what the other people are thinking. A group can go around in circles if everyone is saying, "I don't care" or "whatever" when it's time to make decisions. It can be a leader or a facilitator. One person can serve the role or you can rotate the position.

I like to have clarity in how decisions are going to be made. At the very least, you should talk about group goals and objectives before the trip. Talk about how decisions are going to be made on a day-to-day basis and who will be in charge if there's an emergency. If you talk about these issues, the leadership is more collaborative than if you pretend they don't exist. If you pretend decision making isn't an issue and don't find a good mechanism for it, your group might resort to under-the-table control battles.

**Q:** How should the group choose a leader?

**A:** Leadership isn't anything you do alone—there are all sorts of ways leadership can work in a group. But let's talk about how to choose the person who is going to be the lead architect and leader in, say, an emergency situation or when the group is stuck and needs direction and coordination.

The group members should ask themselves whom they would feel most comfortable taking charge in a difficult situation. That person may be the most competent, the most skilled, the most levelheaded or, likely, a combination of all those qualities. In our society, it's rude to come right out and say, "I'd like to be in charge." But it's worse when no one is willing to step forward until finally the person who does offer to lead ends up being the last person in the world you want leading your group. Have the guts to choose someone good.

**Q:** What leads to breakdown in leadership and expedition behavior in groups?

**A:** Breakdowns usually come when you have no common goals, no common values, and no mechanism for decision making. If your group has a person who wants to lie in the sun and a person who wants to hike 20 miles a day, there has to be a way to work out the differences. Groups and leadership break down far less often, and move past differences more easily, when the objectives and values of the group are understood and accepted by everybody, and when everybody has had a voice in creating them. If I want to sunbathe, I'd be much better off finding a group of sunbathers than trying to turn hard-core hikers on to a sunbathing trip. Birders and photographers figured this out a long time ago—they've formed their own societies. That's not to say groups shouldn't be made up of diverse members—often a wonderful thing—but they need to talk about how they'll work things out.

**Q:** What advice would you give women about leadership in outdoor activities, some of which have long been male-dominated?

**A:** On personal trips, I choose whom I go with and they are always people I want to be around or learn from.

The situation is different if I'm put in a position of leadership and I don't have a choice about the people I'm with. I always try to be myself. I try to see the best in the other group members, male or female. Women offer tremendous qualities in outdoor leadership roles whether or not they're as physically strong as men are. Anyway, many women actually find that what they lack in physical strength, they make up in endurance. Be proud of what you have to offer and learn from others—male and female.

# Leadership

Leadership is a mysterious quality that has baffled historians over the ages. Why can one person with seemingly moderate talents lead a group so well when a person who appears to be his superior in every way fails at the task? Why did Jimmy Carter, a hardworking man with a powerful intellect, have less luck leading Congress than Ronald Reagan, who seemed absentminded and far less concerned with detail? Why do some coaches get so much from a baseball or football team when a coach from just the year before achieved only mediocre results with the same talent pool? If you could identify exactly what makes a good leader and teach it or bottle it, you would probably find yourself in Stockholm accepting a Nobel Prize. Since leadership is a strange combination of chemistry, drive, intelligence, charisma, and circumstance, we can only tilt at what makes it work, why some people have it and others don't, and how to go about developing it in yourself.

Nevertheless, this we know: Leadership matters to the outdoorsperson because expeditions going through the wilds have to make real decisions about real things. Without leadership, the route wouldn't be chosen, the group wouldn't be organized, the pass wouldn't be crossed, and the straggler in the group wouldn't be helped along. What's more, we know that the outdoors is a good environment to learn leadership. The raw quality of traveling in the wilderness forces people to work together and achieve difficult things. Good decisions and good leadership out there are rewarded with tangible success. Bad decisions and leadership go punished. But the results—the cause and effect—are usually clear. The other reason we know that the outdoors is a good place to learn leadership is because we see it in our students over a short month's course. Many a young person starting a NOLS course with next to no visible leadership skills has finished that same course as the chosen leader for his or her small-group expedition.

Over the years, NOLS has identified a set of skills that outdoor leaders should develop and constantly improve upon. Those skills include the following:

▾ Competence
▾ Self-awareness

▾ Judgment and decision making
▾ Tolerance for adversity and uncertainty
▾ Expedition behavior
▾ Communication

**Competence.** The leader of a group does not have to be the best rock climber, map reader, or fisherman, but, all other things being equal, the more competent she is with her technical and organizational skills, the more effective she is likely to be as a leader. People respect competence in leaders for good reason: It suggests self-mastery and a serious approach to the task at hand. And when the going gets tough, competence matters greatly.

**Self-awareness.** You might think of self-awareness as a detached observer or editor sitting on your shoulder keeping you abreast of your moods, your mind-set, and your progress in the world. No person has a perfectly neutral view of himself and the situation at hand, but those with a refined self-awareness come closer to taking an objective view. The self-aware leader has a sense of her prejudices, fears, strengths, and leanings and how those qualities affect her decisions. The leader who knows herself—how she reacts to stress, danger, conflict, and hardship—can adjust to develop a leadership style that suits her accordingly. Self-awareness allows a person to lead without trying to be something she's not.

**Judgment and decision making.** Perhaps the aspect of leadership that Paul Petzoldt most emphasized in developing NOLS is judgment. Petzoldt wrote, "One aspect of leadership is absolute and unquestionable: a leader must be able to make quality decisions, decisions that are based on good judgment, that work, are safe, protect the environment, and accomplish the purpose of the outing."* Judgment is something that can be learned, but only with reflection. Two people who go through the same experience will have two different results. The person who does not reflect on her experience will miss the opportunity to learn and develop her judgment. That person will make the same mistakes over and over and never develop the judgment it takes to be a good leader. The person who takes a moment after a consequential mistake to think things over and reflect on the lesson learned and seek input from outside sources will develop good judgment in a hurry.

Decision making should reflect the gravity and urgency of the decision being made. People naturally like to see decisiveness in their leader. The leader who has a soul-wrenching struggle over the decision of where to stop for

*Petzoldt, op. cit., p. 43.

lunch will not engender much confidence in her group. My brother told me that the time he invests in making a decision is directly proportional to the importance of its outcome—few are the times I've seen him agonize over a breakfast menu. If the choice at hand is of little consequence, your decision should be quick. If the choice at hand bears real importance—the plan to find a missing person—the leader should take reasonable time and involve as many people's ideas as seems warranted.

**Tolerance for adversity and uncertainty.** It's easy being the leader when you're walking down the trail on a beautiful sunny day, the group is full of energy, everyone is healthy, and the birds are singing. But when the group gets lost in a thicket of downed timber, people are fatigued, and the weather is foul, leadership doesn't come easily. Paradoxically, it's these times of adversity when strong leadership is most important. When people feel threatened or uncomfortable, they naturally look for strong leadership. The leader of an outdoor expedition must be mentally prepared to deal with adversity and uncertainty at every turn. Even if she does not have a clear sense of how to solve the problem at hand—be it finding a lost route or managing a medical emergency—being calm and acting deliberately is reassuring to the group. You may have no clue where you are, but you can maintain the group's trust by admitting that and stating a clear plan for getting back on track. Lots of experience with adversity, which comes from lots of experience on outdoor ventures, gives a person the sense of confidence that she can ultimately work with her group and resources to solve the problem at hand.

**Expedition behavior.** We have already discussed expedition behavior at the beginning of this chapter. Good expedition behavior is particularly important for effective leadership. Modeling a high standard of courtesy, selflessness, tolerance, hard work, and flexibility keeps the group standards high.

**Communication.** Good leaders are good communicators. Winston Churchill led England through one of the lowest periods in its history by communicating his conviction that good would ultimately triumph over evil and that the English people would never give up. While your tasks as an outdoor leader are not so difficult as liberating England, good communication may be what gets your group over a high pass or through an interpersonal conflict. To begin, you must let your group know what you expect of them and what they can expect of you. On NOLS courses, we do this the very first day we meet as a group. Instructors lay out the expectations they have for the trip and its members with straightforward standards. It's not easy to get up in front of the group you're leading and say, "This is what I expect of you." Many people assume that if they think the thought hard enough and hint at

## A Designated Leader's Tasks

▾ Prepare and organize.
▾ Let your group know what you expect of them and what they can expect of you.
▾ Stay connected to your group and seek their input.
▾ Use your group's strengths and encourage responsibility.
▾ Take stands on issues clearly and directly.
▾ Work to stay calm and focused.
▾ Endure hardship positively.
▾ Help others when they need it and ask for help when you need it.

what they expect, the team will eventually get the idea and shape up into a well-oiled machine. But it's certainly much more effective, if not more comfortable, to state your expectations and discuss group goals explicitly. If a person on your expedition has made a habit of stealing away with his fishing rod while everyone else sets up camp and prepares dinner, you have a number of choices for how you handle his truancy. You can ignore the person and risk morale problems with the rest of the group. You can give the person dirty looks and make asides under your breath about the person's not helping. Or you can take the person aside, and tell him in frank but polite terms that he is not meeting the group's expectations.

This last approach, while more awkward at the beginning, will usually render the best results.

Leaders need to give their charges feedback often. People naturally like to be told how they're doing in the eyes of the person who's leading. I recently read that the most common reason employees cited for quitting a job is lack of appreciation from the boss. I had assumed that people most often quit their jobs because of money issues or outright abuse. Giving good feedback means being timely (soon after the event at issue and at a time when the person is ready to receive feedback). If you see someone in your group taking a silly risk crossing a river but wait three days to tell her your opinion on the matter, the discussion will lose the good reference of immediacy. Details and context such as the dangers involved and the alternatives are blurred with time.

Good feedback is specific about what it is that the person does well or needs to improve upon. Useful feedback gives a person a very clear idea about what needs changing and steps to make those changes. If someone has an attitude problem because he is not staying warm, dry, and well fed, maybe the simple solution is to give him tips on how to organize his gear and pack so he can take care of himself throughout the day.

Effective feedback is meant to be positive and growth-oriented. Telling the person who crossed the river at the risk of his life that he's a moron and hope-

## Self-Leadership Tasks

▾ Take responsibility for yourself.
▾ Take responsibility for your own learning.
▾ Risk saying what you think.
▾ Own what you say.
▾ If it needs doing, do it.
▾ If you don't understand, ask.
▾ Enjoy your surroundings.
▾ Maintain a sense of humor.
▾ Help others learn and succeed.
▾ Be kind.
▾ Push yourself.
▾ Admit your mistakes.
▾ If it is not safe for the group, don't do it.
▾ Participate and observe.
▾ Learn from your experience.

less isn't feedback but abuse. It doesn't do any good. Effective feedback is oriented at giving people alternatives for the future so they learn and develop judgment (e.g., "next time you come to a river, look downstream and make sure you're not above class-five rapids").

## LEADERSHIP STYLES

Leadership styles depend on both the situation at hand and the personality of the person in charge of the group. Styles range from the very directive—nearly authoritarian—to the entirely consensual, wherein the leader seeks to bring all group members into the decision making through discussion and consultation.

Sometimes it is clear what the problem is and just how it should be solved. A person with a severe head injury needs immediate first aid and prompt evacuation. Such a situation calls for directive leadership, not leadership based on consensus and drawn-out consultation with the group. If the group is caught on a high pass with an approaching lightning storm, it is not the time to circle up the group and chat about the pros and cons of descending versus continuing. Both cases beg for clear and direct leadership. This is not to say that the leader should not draw upon the group as a resource and bounce ideas off her teammates; but it is not a time to worry about whether or not everyone has been included and whether or not a consensual decision has been reached.

Other decisions may be centered around a clear problem or task—how should we plan our route for the trip, perhaps—but with a wider variety of solutions. A clear problem with a variety of possible solutions can be solved either with very direct leadership or with contributions and suggestions from the entire group. The obvious advantage of seeking input from the rest of the group is that members will likely feel more commitment to the decision on how to tackle the problem. What's more, you'll involve more brains and ideas.

Finally, there are times when it's hard to identify the problem and, even more so, the solution. If you have ever directed a play, taught in the classroom, or managed a division of your company, you know that there are times when things aren't going well though you can't put a finger on exactly what the problem is. The group may seem unmotivated, churlish, or low on morale. It's these times that really call for leadership based on discussion and consensus from your group. I suppose the military solution to low morale would be a forced march or more drills, but that hardly works in the world of civilians and certainly not on an outdoor expedition. In many ways, the abstract problems on an expedition are more difficult and demand more art from the leader than the clear-cut medical emergency. I have watched very skilled NOLS instructors adopt a style of leadership that is as subtle as it is effective when group dynamics take a turn for the worse. The leadership involves drawing out the opinions of the entire team, facilitating a discussion, and then working with the group to follow a new direction.

The virtuoso leader can use different styles to meet the problem at hand and has enough experience to know how best to use each style of leadership. In a single day, an outdoor leader may have to take on a direct and even brusque manner with an errant and unsafe climber, delegate tasks, seek consensus and input, and even take on the role of follower during a group discussion. People generally have a style with which they're more comfortable, and some leaders accomplish the same result with a quiet style of leadership as those who use a direct manner. But the broader your repertoire of leadership skills and styles, the more likely you will succeed over the length of the expedition.

# CHAPTER 8

# Maps and Compasses

Just as a good carpenter can envision a complex house—its height, roof pitch, and floor layout—from a set of architectural plans, accomplished outdoorspeople can envision their entire route just from studying maps. Knowing how to read a map well makes planning a route easier: You can better estimate a reasonable day's travel, a good camping spot, and possible evacuation routes. Once out in the backcountry, strong map skills will keep you on your route, or, on the other hand, allow you to deviate from your route to see a special valley or mountain. In an emergency, good map skills make it possible to pinpoint your position so if need be you can alert a rescue party as to your whereabouts. A map is a picture of the world reduced in size thousands of times and then abstracted with colors, symbols, and lines. You might think of it as a blueprint of the backcountry.

If you want to become a capable outdoorsperson, you need to know how to read a map, read the terrain, correlate the two, and navigate your way in varied topography. Camping companies do sell electronic locational devices that can be remarkably accurate, but those can fail and if you lack the map and navigation skill when they do fail, you may find yourself lost, a babe in the woods. What's more, those navigational devices, while they tell you where you are, do not tell you what's ahead.

For the purposes of this book, we will be discussing United States Geological Survey (USGS) contour maps unless otherwise noted.

# The USGS Map

When you first try to read a contour map, you may feel like you are being
given a Rorschach test. To the novice, the colors, symbols, and contour lines
may look labyrinthine and abstract. But give yourself time to learn and before too long, you'll find you can read a map on the basic level.

You will find it easier to understand the section on maps and the section
on compasses in this chapter if you read along with a real USGS map and
compass at your side.

## COLORS

There are six primary colors to a USGS map: green, white, blue, black, red,
and brown. Purple is also used, but used only to delineate revisions.

- ▼ Green represents areas with thick vegetation such as trees and scrub.
  Solid green means the area is forested while the patchwork green means
  the area is covered in scrub.
- ▼ White areas represent areas that do not have significant forests. A typical
  white area would be a meadow, land above timberline, and large gravel
  beds.
- ▼ Blue represents water, be it streams, rivers, lakes, or marshes. Up until
  recently, the solid blue lines showed rivers that run year round while the
  dashed blue lines showed seasonal rivers that only run part of the year.
  But recently the USGS has changed that: Now, a thin blue line represents
  an intermittent stream, while a thicker blue line represents a stream that
  flows year round. Typically these intermittent streams carry water in the
  spring and early summer and then dry up by late summer. Blue also represents contour lines of glaciers and snowfields.
- ▼ Black lines show established trails, light-duty and unimproved roads, and
  management boundaries such as a wilderness area or the division between national forests. Black squares, triangles, and other shapes represent manmade structures such as a cabin or a ranger station.
- ▼ Red lines show U.S. land survey lines, urban areas, and hard-surface
  roads.

▼ The brown lines show the contours of the land and will be discussed below.

▼ Purple lines represent aerial photo revisions that have not yet been field checked.

## SCALE

Maps vary in scale from the overview maps covering hundreds or thousands of miles to detailed maps showing just a few miles. On the bottom margin of your USGS map the scale might be listed as a ratio of 1 to 24,000, for example, meaning that on that particular map, one inch would represent 24,000 inches or two-fifths of a mile of real geography.

USGS cartographers use longitude and latitude to describe the corners and scale of maps. Most USGS maps are of either a 7.5-minute series (1:24,000 scale), 15-minute series (1: 62,500 scale), or a 1 x 2 degree series (1:250,000,000 scale). Truth be told, the USGS is discontinuing the 15-minute map and will soon convert the entire 15-minute series into a 7.5-minute series. A map from the 7.5-minute series covers 7.5 minutes of longitude and 7.5 minutes of latitude. If you hiked from the very northernmost edge of the map to the very southernmost edge, you would hike 7.5 minutes of latitude or about 8.6 miles. Hiking from the easternmost edge to the westernmost edge would take you over 7.5 minutes of longitude. But the mileage covered would depend on how far from the equator you were hiking. In Colorado, crossing 7.5 minutes of longitude would take you across about 7 miles of terrain. Because the lines of longitude are not parallel, USGS maps do not describe perfect rectangles, but rather, quadrangles.

A 7.5-minute map renders lots of detail and can be used to discern subtle changes in terrain. A single map shows an area you might comfortably cross in a single day of hiking, depending, of course, on the terrain and your group.

If you are traveling long distances you may want to carry a planning map drawn to a scale of 1:250,000 in addition to your 7.5-minute maps so you can study the big picture of your route without having to lay out three or four maps on what would undoubtedly be a windy day.

Whenever you're reading a map, keep in mind its scale. Changes in the scale of maps can disorient you. If you are accustomed to using a 7.5-minute map and suddenly switch to a 1 x 2 degree map, remember that what might be a knoll on the 7.5-minute map would be a massif on the bigger map. And what might look like a day's hike on the 7.5-minute map would probably be a couple of days on the other map.

Practice using the scale to judge distances you can see; compare distances you can see with the scale. With some practice you will calibrate your brain to judge distances accurately.

## LATITUDE AND LONGITUDE

If you started in Belem, Brazil (practically on the equator), and flew to the North Pole, you would travel about 6,200 miles or 90 degrees of latitude. Lines of latitude are imaginary lines that begin with the equator and run parallel all the way to the North and South poles. From the equator, there are ninety degrees of latitude to the South Pole and 90 degrees of latitude to the North Pole. Because lines of latitude run parallel to each other, the linear distances measured between degrees are the same: about 69 miles per degree. Every degree is divided into 60 minutes (designated by the symbol ') and every minute into 60 seconds (described by the symbol "). So, one minute of latitude equals 1.15 miles (69 miles divided by 60) and one second of latitude equals about 100 feet.

Lines of longitude divide the world from east to west beginning with zero degrees in Greenwich, England, and going 180 degrees to the date line that runs from the Bering Strait, through the Samoan Islands all the way to New Zealand. The big difference between lines of latitude and lines of longitude is that lines of longitude do not run parallel to each other. They converge on the North and South poles. At the equator, a degree of longitude is equal to 69 miles, but in Colorado, as the lines converge, a degree is only about 50 miles and right next to the North Pole, a degree is only a few feet.

This imaginary grid of longitude and latitude allows us to describe any point on the earth in terms of degrees, minutes, and seconds. Understanding longitude and latitude will help you in map reading and in the use of your compass.

## WHAT'S IN THE MARGINS

- ▾ The top of the map always points north.
- ▾ Map name: Found in the upper right hand and lower right hand corner of the map. Map names usually come from a prominent geographical feature—Hayden Peak, for instance—or from the name of a nearby town.
- ▾ Names of adjoining maps. USGS maps have eight adjoining maps—one on each side and one in each corner. These names (listed in parentheses)

tell you which map you will need to have out as you cross onto the next map.

▼ Longitude and latitude of your map's location. The four corners are each labeled with the longitude (top and bottom of map) and latitude (left and right sides of map) that correspond to their position.

▼ Every 2.5 minutes of longitude and latitude is marked by a fine black line. These can be used to pinpoint your latitudinal and longitudinal location.

▼ Scale: At the bottom center, your map lists the scales as a fraction.

▼ The contour interval: the vertical distance between contour lines.

▼ The direction of true north (represented by the star), the direction of magnetic north (MN), and the declination in degrees between the two. This will be discussed in the section on compasses. (The letters GN stand for grid North Pole, not important for our purposes.)

▼ Date when the map was made and field checked.

▼ Universal Transverse Mercator (UTM) ticks: The UTM system is an international reference system. The distance between blue lines represents a kilometer of distance.

▼ The position of the map in the corresponding state.

▼ The bar scale: This scale gives you a way to calibrate your finger, a piece of string, or a stick to miles, feet, or kilometers.

▼ Key to road symbols.

## CONTOUR LINES

Typical road atlases are two-dimensional because when you're driving a car it's not so important to know the form of the land: Engineers have already built roads that never stray more than 10 percent out of level. But when traveling by foot in the desert canyons or the mountains, a traveler needs to know the shape of the land. She needs to know how steep the passes are so she can figure out how long it will take her to cross them. She needs to know shapes of mountains so she can orient herself and so she can pick a route to the summit. Contour lines give a two-dimensional map its third dimension.

There are several ways to envision contour lines. The most obvious contour lines in the world are the outlines of the continents. Look at the shape of the United States on a world atlas. The coastline that shapes the land from Maine to Florida and from Washington to Oregon is a contour line that delineates sea level.

Contour lines have the following characteristics: They are always level;

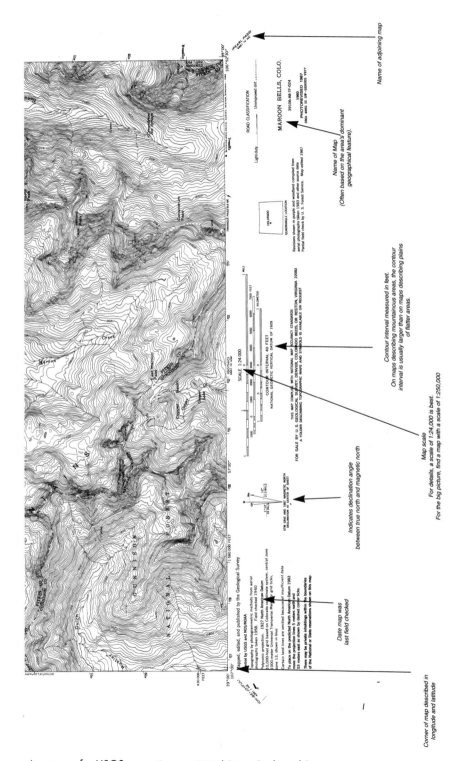

Anatomy of a USGS map. *Courtesy United States Geological Survey*

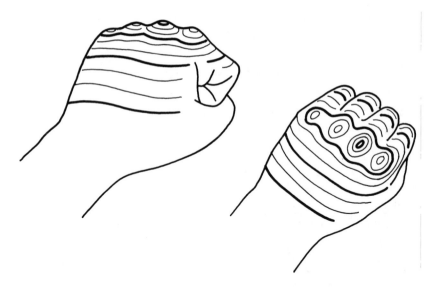

Knuckle mountains. A good way to envision or teach the concept of contour lines is to draw them on a clenched fist, with each knuckle representing a small mountain and the space between knuckles representing saddles.

they are drawn at uniform vertical intervals; and, followed to their end, they form a loop. If you hiked along the side of a perfectly conical volcano at 8,000 feet elevation, neither descending nor ascending, you would eventually end up where you started and your path would trace a circular contour line.

To understand contour lines, fill a glass of water nearly to the brim. The surface of the water at the top of the glass makes a near perfect contour line in the shape of the glass. If you run your hand along the outside of the glass at the surface of the water, your hand will trace a contour line. Your hand is on the same level all the way around the edge of the glass. Now tip the glass about thirty degrees. The shape of the line changes from a circle to an ellipse but you still have a contour line defined by the water surface. The entire oval is at the same level. Still water always finds the level.

Another good way to envision contour lines is to trace the shape of the knuckles on your fist. Make a fist with your nonwriting hand. Hold your fist up to eye level and hold your hand so that your index knuckle is level with the knuckle of your little finger. Now take a pen or marker and make one big circle about an inch from the top of your knuckles at the same level all the way around your knuckles. Next move up about a quarter of an inch and make a line with your pen at the same level. Move up another quarter of an inch and trace another line. This last line will actually end up being four small circles around each knuckle. You now have a contour map of your knuckles. The scale of this map is one to one and the contours represent one-quarter inch of elevation.

As I mentioned before, the brown and dark brown lines represent the contour lines on USGS maps. The contour lines represent regular vertical distances, typically between 20 and 80 feet. Every USGS map has the contour interval listed at the bottom. The contour interval on a flat part of the country—Kansas, say—might be a mere 20 feet. In mountainous Colorado, a map wouldn't have room for all the lines with such a small contour interval.

Every fifth contour line is dark brown and has a number designating the elevation of that particular line. These are called index lines and are very useful for calculating elevation and determining whether your route will be climbing or descending. On a map with a contour interval of 40 feet, the index lines are 200 vertical feet apart (40 × 5).

You should learn to recognize some basic contour shapes and features on your topographical map:

- ▾ A flat area (the contour lines are very far apart)
- ▾ Steep terrain (contour lines very close together)
- ▾ Cliff area (contour lines touching each other)
- ▾ Ridges are shown by a series of V-shaped or U-shaped lines. The apex of the line points downhill.
- ▾ Gullies or couloirs are shaped like ridges but inverted. They are represented by a series of V-shaped or U-shaped lines where the apex of the line points uphill.
- ▾ Saddles, cols, or passes have an hourglass shape that describes a low spot between two higher points. Saddles are important to recognize because they are often the best place to cross a ridge system or mountain pass.
- ▾ Peaks are described by the last circle in a series of concentric circles—sometimes very regular and sometimes oddly shaped. The peak is often designated by an X, a triangle, a number listing the elevation, or a benchmark.

In addition to recognizing these features, it's important to know whether your route will take you uphill or downhill. Refer to the index lines. If your route crosses an index line that says 9,800 followed by an index line that says 10,000, you will be climbing. If your route takes you along a river or stream, you can look at the lines describing it and know your direction of travel that way too. Recall that with rivers, the apex of the V-shape points uphill.

Every fifth contour line is an index line. Index lines list the altitude. They are helpful to determine total elevation gain on your route and to pinpoint your altitude.

Gentle topography as indicated by the large space between contour lines.

Saddle: indicated by hourglass-shaped contour lines.

Very steep slope. The area where the contour lines are touching indicates a cliff.

Perennial stream. A series of V-shaped contour lines indicates the streambed in which the apex of the V's point uphill.

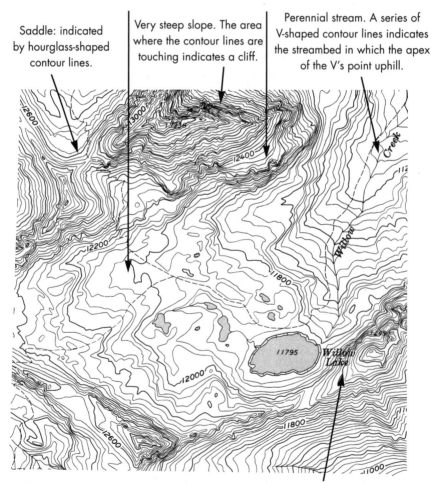

Map topography.

Gentle ridge. Like a streambed, a ridge is described by a series of V-shaped contour lines. But with a ridge, the apex of the V's points downhill.

# Reading Your Map

Many novices new to maps will point to the least likely places when asked to pinpoint their location on a map. They may point to the midpoint on a cliff that Spiderman couldn't scale, when they are in fact in a meadow suited for Julie Andrews and entourage. Until you have played with maps and studied them a bit, you can become confused. It takes a little time and practice to learn to read the topography. To really learn to read the subtleties in terrain from a contour map can take years of practice.

Some people are born with the sort of brain that allows them to rotate strange geometric shapes, a rhombus, say, around a tilted axis, and form a perfect vision of the resulting three-dimensional form—all in their mind's eye. They usually make great map readers and can see things, both on the map and in the real topography, that the rest of us can't. But, above all, everyone can improve their map skills—dramatically—with practice.

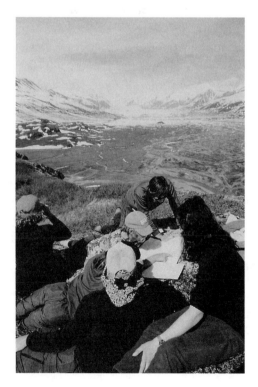

Instructor Tom Haffnor and students check map on an Alaska Mountaineering course. It's easiest to pinpoint your location on a map when you have a clear view of distinct topography such as mountains and rivers.
*Theo Singelis*

## LEARNING TO SEE

To read a map well, we have to learn to see well. Aside from field geologists, surveyors, and mountain guides, few people pay close attention to the lay of the natural world in their ordinary lives. Going about the cities or the interstate systems, we have grids and signs that make the seeing unnecessary. But in the outback, we have to take on the eye of a sketcher and estimate the pitch of a mountain, the distance of a ridge, and the shape of a knoll.

There are really two ways to read a map: One can look at the map first and then try to fit his reading to the terrain about him; or one can look at the terrain first and then try to see where it fits on the map. The second approach, looking at the terrain first, has some real advantages. By studying the terrain without the map you will be able to observe the topography more objectively; you are less likely to make the scene fit some preconceived notion. It's amazing how the mind can interpret and manipulate its reading of the terrain so that it fits the spot where you think you should be on the map—or where you want to be on the map.

There is a constant play between what you see in the real world and imagining how that will look on a map; there is a constant play between looking ahead on the map and imagining what the terrain will look like in real life. By practicing this interpretation of terrain and illustration, you will develop strong map skills.

Start by learning to recognize the most obvious features. Huge pyramidal mountains, knife-shaped ridges, valleys with obvious river bends, and lakes make clear landmarks that you can use to orient yourself. Once you have oriented yourself with an obvious feature, you can then locate more subtle features adjacent to the area. Can you pick out the knoll described by a single contour circle? Can you pinpoint your altitude to within a contour line even on indistinct hillsides? Crossing a series of small, similar drainages, can you pick out which one you're in? Pay attention to every bend in the contour lines and look for the faint changes in pitch, denoted by the contour spacing.

## KEEP YOUR MAP HANDY
## AND KEEP TRACK OF YOUR POSITION

If you have your map in your hands or in a very convenient pocket on your hipbelt, you are much more likely to look at it than if you have to stop and fish around in your pack. Rather than folding and unfolding your map every time you want to look at it, fold it in a way that allows you to see the mile or two you're crossing. A zip-lock plastic bag will keep your map dry and protected for the long haul.

If you start at the trailhead, pinpoint your position on the map (not too hard to do there) and then march the five or ten miles to your camp without looking at your map, you will never develop your map skills. What's more, if you don't keep track of where you are on your map as you travel, it will be that much harder to figure out your location if you get lost.

The good map reader will study his route before leaving camp and then keep track of his position all day. Reading your map and imagining the terrain *before* you hike the next few miles will help keep you oriented. For instance, if you chart a course that begins with 10 ascending contour lines very close to each other, then an area with contour lines that describe a big flat shelf with a marsh in the middle, that's approximately what you should see as you cross that ground. If you hike two hours and haven't climbed at all, you missed your turn. Studying your route on the map first alerts you to what lies ahead.

## ORIENTING YOUR MAP

The first thing to do as a navigator is to orient your map to the real topography that it describes. We will talk about orienting your map with a compass in the next section but it's important to learn to orient your map just by looking at the terrain around you. Why is it important to orient your map? If your map is lined up with the topography it describes, you will find it much easier to read than if you are having to invert features and shapes mentally.

To line up the direction of your map with the real world, you have to find a place where you can see some obvious landmarks. A dense forest is not a good place to orient your map; a broad valley with a river surrounded by towering peaks is a great place to orient your map. One thing to keep in mind as you line up your map is the cardinal directions. Recall that the top of your map should always be pointing north. If you orient your map to the immediate topography around and find that the top of your map is pointing to the early morning sun (east), you are somehow misreading the terrain and need to take another look around you.

Learn to look closely at the features surrounding you. Begin with the most obvious topographical features. Do you see any obvious bodies of water? A large river or a lake? A small stream or a pond? Look at the most dramatic land features. What do the mountains around you look like? Are they towering and snow-capped? Are they rolling hills covered in vegetation? Consider

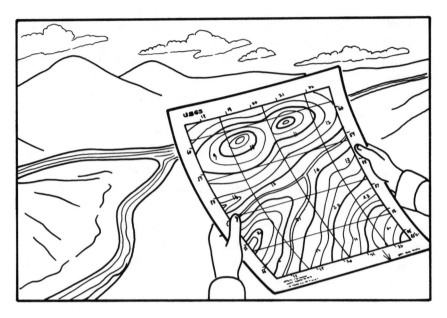

Orienting the map. If possible, find some clearly defined features to orient your map. Rivers, mountains, and valleys are the best. You can orient your map with a compass, but doing it with just the topography is good for your map-reading skills.

the terrain you just crossed. Did you just climb 1,000 feet? Did you just cross a two-mile meadow?

Now imagine a map in your own mind taking into account all these elements. Once you have imagined your map, get out the real map and see if you can find the spot that most resembles what you imagined. Run through your checklist: River to the east? Yes? No? Pyramidal mountain to the south? Large meadow a mile to the west? All the pieces need to fit. You can't be next to a river on your map if there ain't no river where you're standing in the real world.

One of the difficult parts of reading a map has to do with perspective. The maps were drawn using aerial photographs. Normally your view of the world while hiking is from the ground looking up or over. Thus, when you climb a peak or a ridge, your view and likely your accuracy will most closely approach the original survey. If you really feel lost and can't puzzle out how the map fits your surroundings, you may do well to climb to a high point for a bird's-eye view.

Some NOLS instructors teach their students map reading by having them draw their own topographical maps from scratch. It would be a good exercise to develop your own skills. Find a vantage point that gives you a good view of some distinctive topographical features such as a series of peaks or some obvious knolls. Without looking at a map, draw as best you can a section of that topography using contour lines. Compare your drawing to the way the section is presented on an actual USGS map.

## Off-Trail Information

At the bottom of your map you'll see the words "field checked" on a certain date. That date is the last time the area was checked to see if the information on the map was still accurate. What can change? Trails come and go. What looks like an easy-to-follow trail on your map might have been abandoned or forced across a river by an avalanche path. What was once an obvious meadow might be forest now as aspen trees take over. Perhaps the Forest Service has developed a new trail that would change your route planning. If you're hiking in the desert, can you be sure that the watering hole on your map still exists? Might there be places to get water not shown on your map in case of an emergency? Is there a big outfitter's camp you want to steer clear of? You can get this off-trail information from local equipment stores, from the land manager's office, or from talking to friends who know the area.

## Compass

Many associate the compass with navigating the backcountry. They conjure images of ingenious compass work, cracking the puzzle of disorienting terrain. But, in truth, you can do most of your navigating with just a map and an ability to read the topography. The compass is certainly an important tool to the outdoorsperson and something to be mastered. But don't let it become a crutch or your map reading skills will suffer.

The compass is most useful when you don't have distinctive geographical features to orient yourself. Say you're in a flat desert or in a prairie with nebulous terrain. Say you get caught in a whiteout during a snowstorm or on a foggy day. When such terrain or weather makes reading the topography nearly impossible, your compass is most helpful.

The first use of the compass is said to date back to the eleventh century, when people discovered that lodestone, a form of the mineral magnetite, pointed north when dropped in a bowl of water and allowed to settle. Mariners refined the compass by magnetizing a needle and sticking it in a bit of cork or buoyant material. The needle could float freely in water and pointed north. Around the fourteenth century, some clever navigator mounted the needle on the wind rose, a circle divided into sections to distinguish wind directions. Aside from using better materials such as plastic casing, the compass has not changed much since then. A compass today is still a magnetized needle floating in liquid (light petroleum or alcohol) and mounted on a version of the wind rose.

The earth has a magnetic field that runs approximately along its north–south axis. The magnetized needle in your compass will align itself with the earth's magnetic field unless there's something metallic or magnetic that interferes with it. You might think of your compass as a sort of wind vane that always aligns itself with a north-blowing wind.

You will likely find this subject much easier to understand if you have a compass by your side with which to experiment as you read the text.

## COMPASS PARTS

The hiker's compass is a simple instrument. It has the following parts:

- ▼ A free-floating magnetic needle (usually with the north-pointing end colored red)
- ▼ A transparent plastic base plate with a direction-of-travel arrow. Some base plates also have scales in inches or millimeters to help you measure distances on your map.
- ▼ A rotating housing marked with the four cardinal directions (N, S, E, W) and the tick marks representing the 360 degrees of a circle.
- ▼ An orienting arrow drawn on the bottom of the housing (north end often painted red)
- ▼ An index line painted on the base plate. The point where this line meets the tick marks is where you take your compass reading.
- ▼ Some hikers' compasses have a mirror mounted on the base plate to help you sight bearings more accurately.

## DIRECTIONS

As navigators we need a way to communicate precise directions to each other. It would do someone little good if we were to describe a backcountry route by telling them to walk a mile, turn left, walk a mile, and turn right. The cardinal directions—north, south, east, and west—are a little better but still don't allow us the accuracy we need. Thus we have the 360 degrees to describe precisely the direction of travel. Navigators have fixed 0 degrees as

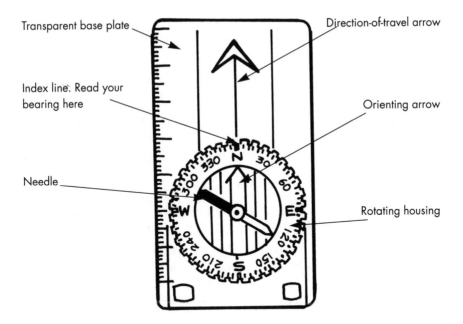

Transparent base plate

Direction-of-travel arrow

Index line. Read your bearing here

Orienting arrow

Needle

Rotating housing

The parts of a compass.

north because north is an easy direction to establish with a compass and at night with the stars. The other cardinal directions are separated by 90 degrees each, going clockwise from north. East is 90 degrees, south is 180 degrees, and west is 270 degrees. With the 360 degrees of direction, we can tell a person to travel on a course of 40 degrees, say, and that person will have much better luck finding the destination than the person told to "head northeast."

## TIPS ON USING YOUR COMPASS

- Make sure your compass is pointing toward the magnetic pole and not toward a local magnetic force or metal object. For instance, if you are standing next to a person who's wearing a giant rodeo belt buckle, your needle may swing in that direction. Hold two compasses close together and watch the needles move around as their magnetic fields influence each other.

- Hold your compass level. For the needle to swing freely, the compass must be kept level. When tilted at a steep angle, the needle can touch the housing and you will not get an accurate reading.

- Check for air bubbles. Leaky compasses get air bubbles under the housing. Air bubbles bigger than about a quarter of an inch can distort the needle's accuracy. At extremely high altitudes, your compass can form air bubbles too.

▼ When taking a bearing, hold the compass at arm's length in front of you. You will get a more accurate reading (analogous to sighting down a rifle).

▼ When adjusting the housing ring, hold the compass close to your body so you can look straight down onto the ring and its index lines.

## BEARINGS

Bearings are simply directions measured in degrees off true north or magnetic north. If true north is described by 0 degrees, then a bearing of 90 degrees describes east and a bearing of 180 degrees describes south. You can take bearings off landmarks and your map, as described below.

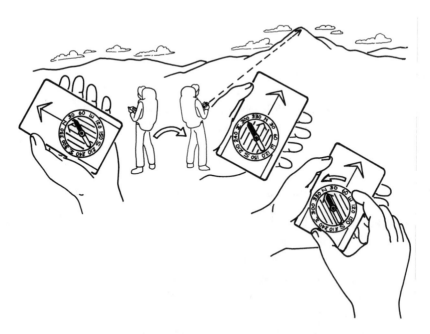

To take a bearing, hold the compass level and in front of you. Turn your body and the compass as one until the direction-of-travel arrow is pointed at the feature you want to measure. Keeping the direction-of-travel arrow pointed at the topographical feature, rotate the housing until the orienting arrow is directly under the magnetic needle. Read your bearing at the index line.

## TAKING A BEARING WITH YOUR COMPASS

Take your compass in hand, and rotate the housing until the N lines up with the index line. Now, holding the compass in front of you—and level—turn your body and the compass as one until the needle is aligned with the orienting arrow. The direction-of-travel arrow is now pointed to magnetic north. Pick a nearby landmark (a tree or mountain, for example) and turn your body and compass together until the direction-of-travel arrow points to the landmark. Keeping the direction-of-travel arrow pointed at the landmark, rotate the housing until the orienting arrow is aligned with the needle (we call this "boxing the needle"). Now you can read the bearing in degrees for that landmark off the index line.

How does this help you in the practical world? Let's say you were standing on a peak with a good view of a lake, where you wanted to camp for the night. Between you and the lake is a dense forest, several undulations in the terrain, and no trail. By taking a bearing of the lake from the peak, and then following that bearing with your compass, you will be able to reach your destination even when you drop down into the forest and lose sight of the lake.

## FOLLOWING A BEARING

It is all but impossible—not to mention awkward and dangerous—to follow a bearing by holding the compass in your hand and keeping the needle lined up with the orienting arrow as you walk across uneven ground. If you are following, say, a 60-degree bearing and stray just a little off your course and then return to your 60-degree direction, you will miss your destination. This is called lateral drift. To follow your bearing accurately, you need to pick intermediate points between you and your destination.

From your starting point take a bearing to your destination. Memorize that bearing or write it down in case your housing rotates accidentally. Now, sighting along the direction-of-travel arrow at your destination, pick an obvious landmark to use as an intermediate point. The intermediate point could be a big tree or an obvious boulder. If the distance to your destination is short, you might just pick one intermediate landmark halfway between you and it. If the distance is far, say three or four miles, you will want to use several intermediate landmarks. Put on your pack, put your compass away, and walk to your intermediate point. But before you go, memorize what your departure point looks like so you can refer to it if necessary (we'll discuss this later). It doesn't matter if you walk to your intermediate point in a straight line or zigzag to get there, and you don't need your compass to get there either.

Once you have arrived at your first intermediate point, take out your compass and make sure that the housing is lined up at the index line to the correct bearing. Box the needle and take another sighting along the direction-of-travel arrow. Pick another intermediate point, put away your compass, and go to the next point. Eventually you'll come to your destination.

In certain situations you may find it impossible to pick a distinct intermediate point. In certain forests, all the trees look alike; a fog may roll in and obliterate the view; or you may be crossing a featureless meadow. When there is no good landmark, use your hiking partner to act as an intermediate point. Have your partner walk ahead a good stretch (but within shouting distance) and while sighting down the compass on your bearing, guide that partner until she is lined up with your direction-of-travel arrow. You and your partner can leapfrog in this fashion until you get to your destination.

## BACK BEARINGS

Back bearings can be used to locate yourself relative to an obvious landmark, to double-check intermediate points, and to find the direction of travel on a return trip. To get a back bearing, you simply add or subtract 180 degrees to the reading at your index line. If the reading at your index line is 180 degrees or more, you subtract 180 degrees to get a back bearing. If the reading at your index line is less than 180 degrees, you add 180 degrees. The back bearing of due east (90 degrees) is 270 degrees (90 + 180) or due west. The back bearing of 290 degrees is 110 degrees (290 minus 180).

If you are standing on a ridge opposite an obvious peak, you can get a rough idea of your location on the map by taking a bearing of the peak and then calculating the back bearing. Say the bearing of the peak from your position is 10 degrees. That means you are on a line extending 190 degrees from the peak (10 + 180). Your location is roughly on the line plotted on your map that comes 190 degrees off the peak and intersects with the ridge you're crossing.

If you used a bearing of, say, 60 degrees to get from a peak to a lake, your return trip to the peak will be the back bearing of 60 degrees, which is 240 degrees. So once you arrive at the lake, you can turn the housing of your compass so the index line reads 240 degrees, box the needle, and make your way back.

Finally, a back bearing can help you determine if you're truly at the correct intermediate point. If you get to your intermediate point—a tree, for exam-

## The Earth's Magnetic Field

Scientists theorize that the earth's magnetic field is caused by the differential in speed between the earth's iron-rich core and the mantle surrounding it. The earth's core rotates slightly faster than the mantle and crust (about one degree per year faster) and acts as a giant dynamo generating a magnetic field.

More important than giving our compasses direction, the magnetic field protects us from cosmic radiation and solar wind. The earth's magnetic field has reversed itself nine times in the last 4,000,000 years. Between reversals, it goes through a sort of transition period wherein the magnetic field is very weak. Scientists don't know the effect on life forms during the periods of low intensity.

ple—and realize that the tree in question looks just like another one 100 feet away, you can take the back bearing of your original course, sight down the direction-of-travel arrow, and you should see your original departure point.

### TRUE NORTH, MAGNETIC NORTH, AND DECLINATION

Magnetic north and the true North Pole are not the same thing. The earth's magnetic field is slightly skewed from the pure north–south axis. However, the difference in direction between magnetic north and true north can be significant enough that you should know how to adjust for it with your compass. The difference measured in degrees between true north and magnetic north is called declination. In a few parts of the world, the direction of true north and magnetic north actually line up and no adjustment for declination is necessary. In the United States, the line of zero declination runs from eastern Minnesota all the way down through Mississippi. But if you travel east of that line to, say, South Carolina, your compass needle no longer points to true north. In South Carolina, the needle points about 6 degrees too far west and therefore has a "westerly declination." If you traveled west from the line of zero declination to, say, eastern New Mexico, your compass would point about 10 degrees too far east—an easterly declination.

Using your map and compass together without compensating for the declination can mean straying way off your intended course. Every five degrees of declination means an error of nearly 500 feet in just one mile's travel. Here in western Colorado, where the declination is 12 degrees, a person who does not compensate for the difference will be over a thousand feet off his route in just one mile of travel.

People new to maps and compasses often get confused about when to adjust for declination with their maps and compasses. But the rule is simple:

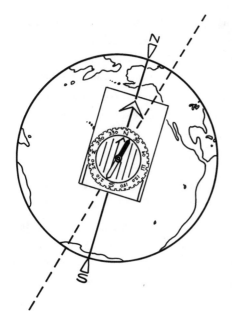

Except in certain states, true north is slightly skewed from magnetic north. USGS maps show the magnetic declination of the area you're visiting in the bottom margin. When using map and compass together, you must adjust for declination or you'll get way off course in short order.

You only have to adjust for declination when the map and compass are being used *together.* If you are using your compass alone to take and follow a bearing, you do not have to adjust for declination.

## ORIENTING YOUR MAP WITH A COMPASS

One of the most useful purposes of a compass is to orient your map. If you come to a pass or an open field with good views of your surroundings, but aren't able to puzzle out the topography, you can use your compass to get your map facing the right direction. To orient your map, follow these steps:

- ▾ Find the magnetic declination listed at the bottom of your USGS map.
- ▾ Turn the compass housing until the number read at the index line corresponds to that declination. For an easterly declination, turn the housing clockwise; for a westerly declination, turn the housing counterclockwise.
- ▾ Place the compass on the edge of the map so that the direction-of-travel arrow is pointing to the top of the map. The edge of the compass needs to be precisely aligned with the left or right edge of the map.
- ▾ Rotate the compass and map together until you have boxed the needle inside the orienting arrow. Your map is now oriented correctly to true

north and the surrounding topography should match what you see on the map. Put rocks or something heavy on the corners of the map to keep it properly aligned.

Though this is a good technique to accurately orient your map, you will develop your map skills faster if you orient the map just by looking at the topography and then checking it with your compass.

### CHARTING A COURSE FROM YOUR MAP

During your trip, you may want to go from your campsite to a lake beyond your line of sight and find that there is no marked trail to the lake. You can find the out-of-sight destination by plotting a course on your map.

- Orient your map with your compass as described above.
- Draw a line between your present position and your destination, using a straight edge.
- Place either edge of the compass on the line you've drawn, with the direction-of-travel arrow pointed at the destination.
- Keeping the compass on the line and the map oriented, rotate the housing until you've boxed the needle with the orienting arrow.
- Read the bearing at the index line. This is the bearing you need to follow to get to your destination.

It may be impossible to get to your destination in just one straight shot. There may be a cliff band or some such obstacle obstructing your route. When that's the case, you will have to break your path up into separate legs and chart the bearings for each leg as described above. Just be sure to pick points at the end of each leg that you can recognize—major knolls, bodies of water, or obvious topographic features. Note how far each leg is so you can have an idea if you've gone too far.

### USING A BASELINE AND AIMING OFF

It's not easy to follow compass bearings with precision. If you are trying to return to your campsite or find a resupply site that is not on a marked trail, it may be easier to aim for a baseline that intersects your destination and then follow that baseline to where you want to go. A baseline is any topographic feature that runs an easy-to-follow course. A baseline could be a river, a road, or an obvious ridge that would be easy to keep in sight and follow.

Say you're returning from a day hike and know your campsite is on a major river. Rather than trying to follow a bearing precisely to your campsite, you can just aim for the baseline—the river in this case—and then follow it to your camp. The only complication is this: How do you know what direction to turn once you hit the baseline? The solution is to deliberately "aim off" a little when you plot your course. If the river runs east to west, you could aim off by plotting a course that takes you too far east of your destination. Then, once you hit the river, you simply follow it on its westerly course.

# Navigation

When you travel in popular areas that have well-marked trails, route finding is easy. Certain parts of Yosemite, Yellowstone, and Rocky Mountain National Park have trails so well traveled and so well marked that getting from point A to point B is no more difficult than finding a gate at the airport. But if you travel in less known areas where even trails marked on the map fade away every few miles, route finding will test your skills. If you decide to go off trail, whether it's to see new areas or to take a shortcut, your navigational skills will decide whether indeed you come out the other side.

Just reading this chapter and spending a short week in the mountains is not enough to give you excellent navigational skills. It takes time and miles and mistakes to learn how to pick your way through the backcountry. As with any art, you can spend a lifetime learning how to get better at it.

Route finding is part map reading and part instinct. Perhaps the most important principle is to always keep a sense of the big picture. Novices tend to lose sight of the greater surroundings as they focus on their map and the trail at their feet. Many a novice NOLS student will take out a map in the thickest, darkest bushes hoping for clues as to their location. But the map will tell you nothing if you don't have topographical context. Likewise, novices can become flustered at an unmapped fork in the trail even if the topography— a deep narrow valley, for instance—suggests that the trails have to meet again soon.

# Time Control Plans

At NOLS we teach students to write Time Control Plans (TCPs). A TCP is simply a detailed itinerary of the day ahead. Writing TCPs forces you to look closely at the route, anticipate the terrain and obstacles in advance, and helps you create a mental picture of the route before you get there. Writing TCPs teaches map-reading skills, route planning, and orients you to the terrain you will cross.

Whether you write a TCP or not is of course up to you. The detail of the TCP is also up to you. But do consider at least the rudiments. Trying to envision the route ahead will help develop your map and navigation skills and will help you get to your destination as well.

A TCP includes the following information:

▾ Group Information including: Number of people in group. Name of the group leader. Group gear (such as tent, stove, first aid equipment, etc.).

▾ Starting point: Geographical description of starting point including longitude and latitude, common name.

▾ Destination: Geographical description of your destination including longitude and latitude and common name.

▾ Distance to be traveled: Try to estimate this distance to within a half-mile accuracy. Remember to look at the switchbacks.

▾ Elevation gained: Calculate the total elevation you will *gain* in the day. Say you climb 2,000 feet up a pass and then drop down 1,000 feet and then climb 500 feet up to the top of another pass. The total elevation, then, is 2,000 feet plus 500 feet for a total of 2,500 feet (elevation descended is not included in the calculation because it is usually the climbing that really changes your pace on the trail). For every 1,000 feet you have to climb, add a mile to your travel time.

▾ Time: Estimate your travel time by looking at the terrain ahead of you. Is it difficult terrain or rolling meadows? Will you be on a trail or traveling off trail? How heavy are your packs? Do you have to cross rivers? What is the health of the group? Are there any injuries that will slow the group down? Typically you can travel between one and two miles per hour (including rest breaks) when backpacking. If your whole team is very fit, you can travel faster than that.

▾ Description of route: Your description should describe in detail the terrain you anticipate crossing, major topographical features you will pass (mountains, passes, rivers, etc.). The description should go beyond simply saying "We will follow the Glacier trail for ten miles until we come to Blue Lake." Pretend there is no trail and you have to describe your route so that someone searching for your party could find you just by the landmarks you list.

▾ Contingency plan: The contingency plan forces you to think about the "what ifs." What will you do if you can't make it to your campsite?

Where will you camp instead? If you are in the desert, will there be water? If you are in the mountains, will there be sufficient shelter? What if
a lightning storm keeps you from crossing a pass? What if you can't cross
the river along your route?

▼ Obstacles and hazards: What do you see on the map or in the sky that
could trip you up? Do you have a 12,000-foot pass to cross? Are there
threatening clouds to the west? Do you have to cross a river? Have you
been told that the trail has a lot of downed timber?

TCPs are also useful to leave in town with others so that they might more
easily find you in the case of an emergency, especially if you are traveling
solo.

# Tips on Route Finding

## Hand Rails

Hand rails are topographical features that you can use to stay on course.
A rail might be a river or a ridge. Even the sun can act as a rail. For instance,
if you know that you are traveling from east to west, you know that you're in
the Northern Hemisphere and it's late summer, then you should know approximately where the sun should be relative to you throughout the day. In
the morning it should be behind you. At midday it should be overhead but
slightly to your left (south), and in the afternoon it should be in front of you.
If you are an hour into the day and the trail takes you through a thick forest
and suddenly you come out and are facing the sun, something went wrong.

# CHAPTER 9

# Emergency Procedures

I watched a movie last night about three very urban men stranded in the mountains of Alaska after a plane accident. Despite surviving the crash intact, things turned nasty right away as a giant grizzly began stalking them. Before long, the bear dined on one of the unfortunate men.

Over the course of a few days, the remaining two men managed to kill the bear with a fire-hardened spear, fashion some rather spiffy outfits from the bear's hide, cross treacherous mountains and rivers, and still have enough energy to come to blows over a woman back in the city. Survival!

I thought about the movie and compared it to a conversation I had with John Gookin, NOLS director of curriculum and resident brain. When I asked John what sort of equipment he would include in a survival kit, he said a waterproof lighter, a small compass, a small whistle, and a water bottle. Having a lighter, compass, and whistle along makes obvious sense, but why the water bottle? "The best tool you have for a survival situation is your brain," Gookin said, "and keeping your brain hydrated is key to clear thinking." Gookin had some good tips for survival situations, but the gist of his ideas centered around deliberate decision making, calm thinking, and using judgment. I think if John had written the plot for the survival movie it would have been pretty dull stuff: three guys drinking water, talking things through, trying not to aggravate the darn grizzly bear, and probably coming out of the woods in awfully good shape—sans the snazzy bearskin outfits. In John's movie, I guess the men would have followed the low Alaskan sun—practically begging them to head south—instead of making their own compass from a paper clip (and wandering in circles), would have tried to find an easier river crossing than the raging torrent the men in the movie crossed, and might have even come to a peaceful solution over the woman. But that's why John's in Lander, Wyoming, training NOLS instructors instead of making blockbusters in Hollywood.

In his book, *The New Wilderness Handbook,* Paul Petzoldt titled the second chapter not "Survival" but, rather, "Avoiding Survival Situations." The chapter begins, "Avoidance of a survival situation is more important than learning how to get out of a survival situation." If you ever take a NOLS course, chances are your instructors will put more emphasis on teaching you to plan well, to think things through, and to develop good judgment than they will on teaching you how to clean up wilderness disasters. The philosophy at NOLS centers around living comfortably in the outdoors based on self-reliance, thoughtful action, and skills, not on waging an epic battle against Mother Nature and the stoutest of her critters.

If you plan your trip well, bring good equipment, practice leadership and good expedition behavior, and use your head and good judgment out there, you will probably not get yourself into a survival or emergency situation. Having said that, you should plan your trip and your training with the assumption that you *will* have to deal with an emergency. To be a capable outdoorsperson, you should learn at least basic wilderness first aid and preferably advanced wilderness first aid. I say *wilderness* first aid because while many of the principles are the same as standard "urban first aid," a remote setting will force you to use your wits, improvise, provide extended care, and plan more thoughtfully. Whereas your best response to, say, a fallen skateboarder in downtown Los Angeles might be to stabilize the victim and then call 911 and wait for the ambulance to show up, you don't have that luxury while out camping in the backcountry. You shouldn't assume that you can radio for help and cool your heels while the helicopter flies in—deus ex machina—to scoop up your injured friend. First of all, even if you are carrying a cellular phone or a radio, you may be out of range or your batteries can die. Second, poor weather and visibility might make it impossible for a helicopter to land at the accident site. Finally, self-sufficiency is part of the outdoor ethic. Think of your party as a self-contained unit that depends on no one. You will plan better with that mind-set, travel more sensibly, and be less likely to get into a wreck. Helicopter evacuations are major ordeals: expensive, dangerous, and intrusive on the wilderness—even embarrassing. They're not always a possibility either. In less developed countries, the local township simply may not have the big bird, no matter your predicament. In any event, you should only call for a helicopter in dire situations as discussed below.

The difficulty of evacuating a full-sized adult should impress upon you the need to be more conservative in the outback. The financial costs and environmental impacts are significant. This chapter discusses some emergency procedures, the planning and executing of an evacuation, searching for lost party members, and staying found.

## Emergency Procedures

Time takes a strange warp when you are faced with a medical emergency. For some, a crisis calms the mind to a point where they think clearly and act deliberately. These people usually make sensible plans for handling the injured party. The important thing to remember about time in the backcountry is that once you have stabilized the scene—stopped the bleeding, treated for shock, or resuscitated the victim—rushing to send a messenger team or launch the evacuation will probably make little difference on the positive side and could lead to botched plans. Will a twenty-minute head start really make a difference in a ten- or twenty-hour evacuation? Probably not. Will twenty minutes of extra planning and thought before sending a messenger team really make a positive difference? Probably yes.

At NOLS, there is an old saying about what to do when pressed with an emergency: "Stop and smoke a cigarette." The saying is obviously not meant to be taken literally but rather as a way to remember to think things through. Stanching the blood flow of a wounded person obviously calls for quick action and little reflection; but planning what to do after you have performed the basic first aid calls for the metaphorical cigarette.

### WHEN TO EVACUATE
### AN INJURED OR SICK GROUP MEMBER

The decision whether or not to evacuate a victim depends on the severity of the injury or illness. In most cases it really depends on the patient's ability to participate in the expedition and the expedition members' willingness to accommodate an ill or injured party member.

The decision to evacuate a patient should not be taken lightly. At the very least, it may disrupt or end a long-planned trip. Worse, it can place your group and the rescuers at risk: Litter carrying is very hard work; helicopters crash.

Patients usually fall into one of three categories. First, there are those who have obvious and severe injuries such as head injuries, signs and symptoms of a heart attack, or severe abdominal pain. Such illnesses and injuries are usually easy to spot, and the need for evacuation is obvious. Second, there are injuries and illnesses that are not life threatening but nevertheless prevent a person from participating in the trip. These include (but are not limited to) sprains, broken teeth, mild diarrhea, or the flu. Finally, there are patients with signs and symptoms that are difficult to interpret. You'll scratch your head and wonder if they need to see a doctor or if it's safe to keep them on the expedition.

The best way to be prepared for all three of these cases is to have training in wilderness first aid (a subject that is a book unto itself). This training is important to your backcountry skills and certainly something that will help you when you need to decide whether or not one of your party members needs to be evacuated.

## STEPS TO A SAFE EVACUATION

Delegate roles and responsibilities: If you are the team leader, you need to give yourself the time and space to think and act as leader. Don't attempt to stabilize the victim, take first aid notes, pitch the tent, and plan an evacuation by yourself or you'll be so focused on tasks that you won't be able to look at the big picture. Choose a clear role for every member of your team depending on his or her experience, demeanor, and state of mind. Imagining a hypothetical emergency in advance will help you consider the strengths and weaknesses of your teammates before you have to assign roles. Even if you only need one or two people to secure the scene, find chores for the other members of the group. Purposeful action will help them feel involved and stay calm. Nonessential but useful chores might include heating water for hot drinks, setting up a tent, and locating the party's position on a map.

## EVACUATION OPTIONS

There are two primary options to consider in the event that you decide to perform an evacuation: self-rescue/evacuation or assisted rescue/evacuation. There are a number of factors to consider in deciding whether you can perform a self-rescue or need outside assistance. These factors may include but are not limited to the following:

- ▾ Severity of the injury or illness
- ▾ Whether or not the patient can walk

▾ Physical strength of the group
▾ Number of people in your party
▾ Skills and ability of the group to conduct a litter evacuation
▾ Willingness of the group to do the evacuation work and accept the disruption to the trip
▾ Distance to the roadhead
▾ Difficulty of the terrain
▾ Weather conditions
▾ Communications options
▾ Available assistance

### Self-Rescue/Evacuation

How do you know if the lamed can get out on his own? An old saying goes "If you can walk, you can walk." The injured person's reaction to walking is likely your best way to judge whether he or she needs to be carried out or can get out on their own. Someone with a moderate sprain can probably walk to the road if the rest of the group carries his pack weight. You may have to build him a makeshift crutch or cane or give him bodily support. Creativity and ingenuity may be necessary to negotiate certain obstacles. You may have to piggyback him across a river or creek and he may need to crab-walk across a short boulder field, talus slope, or steep section of the trail.

Carrying the patient out on a litter should be considered if the patient cannot walk and medical attention can be delayed by 24 hours or more. Many types of litters can be constructed using trees, climbing ropes, backpacks, and other equipment you have on a backpacking trip. The NOLS Wilderness First Aid book covers this subject in detail. Two key factors to consider when deciding whether or not to carry a litter are the difficulty of the terrain and the strength of your group. If you are a group of three, including the downed member, and ten treacherous miles from the nearest road, this is obviously not a good choice. You simply don't have the manpower. But if you are, say, a group of six strong people, the downed member is not some retired sumo wonder, and you are not an impossible distance from a road, you can with some toil and sweat haul him or her out to medical help.

### When to Seek Outside Assistance

If self-rescue is not feasible, you will need help from others. Help might come from a local search and rescue team, a local law enforcement agency, public land management agencies, or other backcountry travelers in the nearby area. Options that may be available include helicopters, additional manpower to carry a litter, or horsepackers (in cases when the patient is able to ride a horse).

Contacting outside assistance requires some form of communication such as a cellular phone or satellite phone or a radio. Obviously you need to know the phone numbers or the radio frequencies of those you want to contact before you leave for the backcountry. Remember the limitations of these electronic devices as discussed earlier.

A reliable but slower method of getting outside assistance is to send messengers—two or three people from your group who hike out to a phone or ranger station to request help.

No matter how you request help, you need to be carefully prepared with the following:

1. Prepare a written message that is concise and to the point. A written message reminds the person using a cell phone or radio to include all the pertinent information in a logical manner. Likewise, the written message helps the messenger remember important details such as location of the accident site. The message should include the number of injured; the patient's name, age, and gender; location of the patient; description of the accident or illness; mechanism of injury; the patient's current condition; a description of the first aid provided and other medical notes; and whether or not you need an EMT or paramedic.

2. Identify your location on a map. The best method for identifying your location is to use latitude and longitude (see Chapter 8). It is more accurate in many cases than a written description of the site, and most reputable search and rescue groups use latitude and longitude routinely. Include the name of the USGS map that shows where the patient is and any common names of nearby topography. If sending messengers, send a set of maps marked with the location of the patient and the route taken out of the backcountry. It is vital that you get this information right because search and rescue teams will need this information to find the patient.

3. When sending a messenger team, write out a plan that includes: what roadhead they will go to; phone numbers they will need; who they will attempt to contact once they reach the phone; what the patient's group will do (normally it will wait, but sometimes it will have to move to a more suitable site); what the messenger team will do once it reaches help; a contingency plan in case the messenger team is delayed or doesn't make it to the roadhead; and how the messenger team will rejoin the main group.

4. Messenger teams need to be able to travel quickly but should be prepared to spend one or two nights out. They may also need to be prepared to camp at the roadhead while waiting for help to arrive. Consequently, they should carry food, shelter, a stove, fuel, cookware, and warm clothes. When selecting a messenger team, include your strongest hikers and best map readers. If you have the resources, a team of four is considered the best number. Should one of the team be injured, one person can remain with the injured party while the other two continue for help. Messengers need to hike quickly but not so hastily that they risk injuring themselves.

## IF YOU REQUEST A HELICOPTER

Theoretically, sending for a helicopter is something to do only in a dire emergency such as a life-threatening injury or illness, or in the event that the patient is in a condition too delicate to be carried out by other means. The reality, however, is that in parts of the country, including the Rocky Mountain West, search and rescue teams use helicopters for less serious cases. When the weather is right, a helicopter is fast and efficient and often easier than organizing a rescue team. Even if you don't request a helicopter when you send your messenger team, have a landing site prepared in case the local authorities choose to send one.

### Preparing for a Helicopter Landing

- ▾ Provide a wind direction indicator such as a brightly colored shirt or ground cloth tied securely to a tree.
- ▾ Find a site that is at least 100 feet in diameter and preferably one that allows the helicopter an approach and takeoff from 360 degrees. If possible the site should allow the helicopter to land at an approach angle of as low as 15 degrees.
- ▾ Mark the landing site with a large bright X that can sustain the 200 mph winds generated by the helicopter.
- ▾ Remove all loose debris and equipment within 100 feet of the touchdown site. Loose objects can be sucked into the helicopter's rotors and cause a crash.
- ▾ Help the pilot identify the site by standing at least 100 feet from the landing area with your back to the wind and your arms extended in the direction of the landing area. Wear eye protection.
- ▾ Do not approach the landed helicopter until the pilot indicates it is safe to do so. Keep your head down and approach the helicopter from the

downhill side to stay beneath the rotors. Always stay in the pilot's view. Never approach the helicopter from the rear or you could walk right into the rear rotor.

# Search and Rescue

## FINDING THE LOST PERSON

When you first discover that one of the group members is lost, your instinct may be to go tearing off in the direction you last saw the person, shouting their name. If everyone in your group has the same instinct, the list of lost persons may soon include the entire group. If ever there is a time that triggers panic, it is when someone gets lost. But if ever there is a time when you need to stay calm, think clearly, and act deliberately, it is at the very time when your inner voice may be screaming "Freak out!" The good news is that lost people are usually found.

### Steps to Take When a Person in Your Party Gets Lost

▼ Mark your map with a *point last seen* (PLS). This is the point where you actually saw the person last, not where you guess he or she might have gone.

▼ Mark any clues on the map, but don't use them to shift your PLS unless you're absolutely certain of your clue. Clues might include the direction you last saw the person walking, a comment or conversation (e.g., the person told you he or she really wanted to go fishing alone), a chore that would require the person to walk in a certain direction (e.g., fetching water).

▼ Quickly set up some kind of confinement in order to keep the person in the area. This could include leaving notes at trail intersections or roadheads, or placing sleeping bags, bonfires and other attraction devices on prominent points. Many lost people are found by confinement. Confine quickly and about twice as far out as you think the lost person has wandered.

▼ Send an initial response team to any likely accident sites. When you have limited searchers, you are more concerned with looking for an accident scenario than you are in finding people who have simply strayed off. Use your intuition and map-reading skills to decide where to send your initial response teams. More often than not, lost people stray downhill, sometimes really far downhill. They usually don't accidentally climb

very high. Accident sites might include steep riverbanks, stream crossings, bear hangs, and steep slopes.

▼ From your PLS on your map, draw a circle with a radius three miles out,
then draw a second circle with a radius of six miles out. Statistically, half
of all lost people will be found in the first circle, 90 percent within the
larger circle.

▼ Divide the search area into segments defined by obvious barriers or landmarks such as a river, a ridge, or a lakeshore. Record your search efforts.

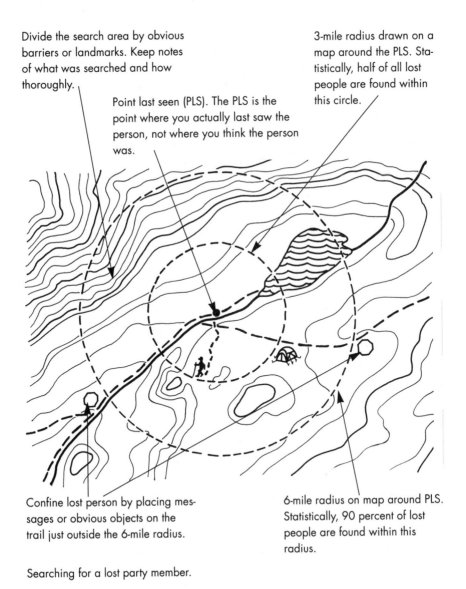

Divide the search area by obvious
barriers or landmarks. Keep notes
of what was searched and how
thoroughly.

3-mile radius drawn on a
map around the PLS. Sta-
tistically, half of all lost
people are found within
this circle.

Point last seen (PLS). The PLS is the
point where you actually last saw the
person, not where you think the person
was.

Confine lost person by placing mes-
sages or obvious objects on the
trail just outside the 6-mile radius.

6-mile radius on map around PLS.
Statistically, 90 percent of lost
people are found within this
radius.

Searching for a lost party member.

Mark the map to show where you checked and keep notes regarding how thorough the search was. These notes will provide critical data should the search last for more than a day or two. Without detailed information, future searches will merely duplicate your efforts.

Here are some tips that save time in finding people:

- Mobilize fast if you suspect an injury or illness.
- Send your best searchers to the areas most likely to contain the lost person.
- Advise your search teams to travel light: They are search teams, not rescue teams.
- Search for clues, not just the subject. If you go tearing down the trail looking for the lost person, you may miss important clues along the way such as broken branches, footprints, or an unmarked fork in the trail.
- Skip grid searches; statistically, they're a waste of time.
- Don't forget that lost people sometimes move back into places where you already looked.
- Operate at night only if it is a crisis; night searches wear people out and are inefficient.
- Expect it to take a half-day for the search and rescue team to mobilize a significant force. With this in mind, it is better to call for help a little early rather than a little late.
- The following factors can affect the situation's urgency: the person's age, fitness, mental state, clothing, skills, special medical concerns, the current weather, predicted weather, terrain, altitude, the strength of your group, and your intuition.

### GETTING FOUND

Just as a lost person can inspire panic in a search party, getting lost yourself may tempt you to abandon your reasoning faculties, rush about the mountains with little thought, and get yourself still more lost. If you get lost, you would do well to consider the above advice for the searchers and apply all the corollaries:

- A good search and rescue team will concentrate on the PLS and the circle within a three-mile radius. Ergo, stay in the vicinity of where you first realized you were disoriented. If you do explore possible routes back to camp, take a tip from Hansel and Gretel, look back a lot and mark your trail so you can backtrack to your last point. Make arrows showing the direction in which you are traveling.

▼ Conserve energy by resting when you can.

▼ Look for ways to signal for help, including hanging bright objects, building smoky fires, and making noise. A signal mirror is from 10 to 100 times more visible than any other object.

▼ Wander out a short distance (no more than a quarter of a mile) from the spot where you're waiting and place markers pointing to your spot. Use rocks, broken branches, dirt, or anything else you can arrange into a geometric pattern. Geometric patterns—triangles, squares, and circles—are easier for searchers to notice than most other attraction devices.

## TIPS ON SURVIVING IF YOU GET SEPARATED FROM YOUR GEAR OR GROUP

▼ Stay hydrated. Without water, your thinking will be muddled within 12 hours.

▼ Take a nap during the day when it is warmer because chances are you won't sleep well at night without a sleeping bag, pad, and tent.

▼ If you are hiking, stop early in the afternoon at a site with water and cover.

▼ When you stop for the night, do everything possible to stay warm. Build a fire if possible. Put on all your layers—even your sunglasses will help prevent heat loss from around your eyes. You can stuff leaves and pine needles under your outer shell for added insulation. Find something to insulate you from the ground: pine needles, climbing ropes, your internal frame pack, etc.

▼ In hot climates avoid heat exhaustion by traveling only in the early morning or later in the afternoon. During the hottest part of the day, protect yourself in the shade.

▼ Remember, you can go a week without food and remain quite healthy. But it is harder to stay warm without regular meals. The problems associated with the first week without food are more psychological than physical.

# What's in Buck's First Aid Kit

Buck Tilton is cofounder of the Wilderness Medicine Institute, one of the leading teachers and sources of wilderness medicine. He is author or coauthor of 17 books, most of them dealing with wilderness medicine and rescue. Here is what he carries in a typical first aid kit when he goes backpacking:

▾ Rubber gloves: to prevent contamination from body fluids.
▾ Pocket rescue mask: to avoid contact with body fluids during rescue breathing.
▾ Irrigation syringe: the best device for cleaning wounds.
▾ Antibiotic ointment: to cover small wounds once they've been cleaned.
▾ Adhesive strips (e.g., Band-Aids).
▾ Sterile gauze pads and/or sterile rolls of gauze: for cleaning and covering wounds. Roll gauze can also hold splints in place.
▾ Athletic tape (1 inch by 10 yards): It holds down the gauze, prevents blisters when applied to sensitive spots at the start of a trip, and repairs injured equipment for short periods of time. Athletic tape shapes itself more easily to the strange designs of human extremities and can be used to wrap ankles supportively.
▾ Tincture of benzoin compound: Benzoin rubbed on skin helps things with adhesive such as athletic tape or moleskin stick better. This is particularly helpful if you have dirty, sweaty skin.
▾ Wound closure strips: for pulling together the sides of a clean, gaping wound.
▾ Microthin film dressing (e.g., Opsite): to cover cleaned wounds.
▾ Molefoam and/or 2nd Skin: These work great to prevent blisters if applied before the damage is done. Use them to treat blisters after a bubble has developed.
▾ Soap-impregnated sponges (e.g., green soap): for cleaning wounds.
▾ Elastic wrap and/or Coban: can be used to compress strains and sprains for a little added comfort, or used to hold a possible broken bone to a splint, or used to hold a bulky dressing on a bad bleed, or used in any other creative way you can think of.
▾ Trauma shears: very strong scissors for cutting up just about anything.
▾ Tweezers (forceps): for removing splinters, etc.
▾ Safety pins: They can secure the elastic wrap, be sterilized and puncture a blister to drain it, repair rips in clothing.
▾ Painkiller: Buck prefers ibuprofen because it's an anti-inflammatory as well as a pain reducer. This medication can bring a bit of relief after you have grown a headache, a muscle or joint ache, or just about anything that causes painful discomfort. And it reduces a fever.
▾ Antihistamine tablets: Benadryl is probably the best for most people's allergies. Their sedative effect helps relieve the itch of allergies and insect bites, helps you get to sleep (so don't take one and continue a high risk outdoor activity), and helps ease the symptoms of a cold.
▾ Imodium: for diarrhea.

# CHAPTER 10

# Weather

Even with the best minds and the biggest computers, scientists cannot predict the weather beyond three or four days with much accuracy. There are too many variables. Long-term weather forecasting may never be possible because of the chaotic nature of the atmosphere. In 1960, the meteorologist Edward Lorenz discovered that complex mathematical equations rendered radically different results when one of the variables was altered only slightly. Since weather forecasting is largely a giant mathematical model with millions of variables, Lorenz determined that long-term forecasts could never be done with any sort of accuracy. He concluded that something as insignificant as the beating of a butterfly's wings in Peru could radically change the weather in Texas. But that's part of the great adventure of the outdoors. Things would be awfully dull if the temperature stayed at 60 degrees, the sky kept its azure color, and the clouds were just soft cotton balls wandering aimlessly across the sky. Even if we try to stay clear of the storms when we're out camping, the threat of dark clouds, a brisk wind, and the drama of a good lightning show gives our expedition its Sturm und Drang.

In his bestselling book *Into Thin Air,* Jon Krakauer captures the mystery of weather with one chilling paragraph:

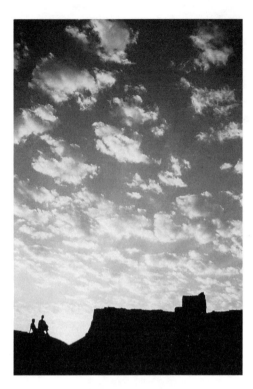

Weather: Hope for the best, but don't get lulled by blue skies. With weather it's best to be flexible with your plans and to try to take advantage of local and seasonal atmospheric patterns. These are cumulus clouds. *Chris Myers*

I can attest that nothing I saw early on the afternoon of May 10 suggested that a murderous storm was bearing down. To my oxygen-depleted mind, the clouds drifting up the grand valley known as the Western cwm looked innocuous, wispy, insubstantial. Gleaming in the brilliant midday sun, they appeared no different from the harmless puffs of convection condensation that rose from the valley almost every afternoon.

Weather is capricious but every area of the world has its atmospheric extremes and disposition. Where I live here in the Colorado Rockies, the cumulonimbus clouds march out of the west nearly every summer afternoon and form awesome thunderheads. Not all these towering clouds develop lightning and thunder, but many do. In this area, we time our peak ascents with early morning starts so we can beat the afternoon's thunderheads. In Mexico's Baja California, NOLS sea kayaking courses are ever watchful of "El Norte," a strong wind that comes out of the north and roughs up the sea. In your expedition planning, you would save yourself unpleasant surprises by learning the weather patterns of the area you're visiting.

Beyond that, we can look at the sky for signs of advancing weather to make short-term forecasts (i.e., within 24 hours). Just knowing the basics of weather mechanics, understanding some of the more obvious signs, and paying attention to the sky can help you make an educated guess as to what's coming in your direction. In that way, you can take advantage of the clear days, or, on the other hand, batten down the tent for a storm.

# Clouds

Not including the use of instruments, clouds give us the most information about approaching weather. A variety of stratus and cirrus clouds arriving in a certain order announce the approach of a warm front and possibly several days of precipitation. The ominous lenticular cloud positioned over a high peak tells the eager climber to wait a day or more for the winds to die down.

In the early 1800s, an English meteorologist by the name of Luke Howard devised a classification of clouds based on their shape, the distance they floated from the earth, and whether or not they were rain-producing. Howard used Latin names to describe these clouds and his taxonomy is still in use today. He identified the following three shapes:

- ▾ **Cirrus** (Latin for "curl of hair"), which are stringy, fibrous clouds.
- ▾ **Cumulus** (Latin for "heap"), which are puffy clouds that frequently resemble a cotton ball. They have a lot of vertical dimension (i.e., are as tall as they are long) and float through the sky separate from each other.
- ▾ **Stratus** (Latin for "layer"), which are clouds that form long bands and layers, sometimes covering hundreds of thousands of square miles.

Howard came up with just two classifications for the height at which clouds float above the earth:

- ▾ **Cirro,** which refers to clouds whose base begins at or above 20,000 feet.
- ▾ **Alto,** which refers to clouds whose base begins somewhere between 6,000 and 20,000 feet.

Finally, Howard used the term **nimbo** (as a prefix) or **nimbus** (as a suffix) to describe rain-producing clouds. These Latinate terms can be used separately or combined to describe any cloud you see in the sky.

Figure 10-1 summarizes the ten basic cloud types. Most of these clouds are easy to identify in the sky. Looking at just one cloud in the sky may tell us little about the weather; but watching a series of different cloud formations develop over a period of hours or days can warn of impending fronts.

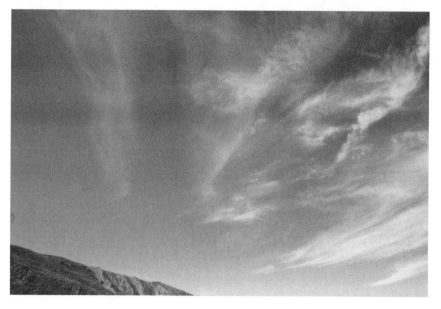

Cirrus clouds are thin and wispy. They usually form above 20,000 feet and move from west to east in alignment with the prevailing upper winds. *Mark Harvey*

## Air Masses and Fronts

When a huge body of air (big enough to cover several states) stays in one place for a week or two, it develops uniform qualities of temperature and humidity that match the ground or ocean below it. Air that stays over Alaska for several days becomes dry and cold. Air that stays over the Gulf of Mexico becomes warm and moist. There are four basic air masses that affect weather in the United States:

- ▾ **Continental polar air masses.** Air masses that originate over Alaska and northern Canada.
- ▾ **Maritime polar air masses** begin over the northern oceans and are cool and humid (though warmer than continental polar air masses).
- ▾ **Maritime tropical air masses** form over the Gulf of Mexico and the Caribbean. They are warm and moist.
- ▾ **Continental tropical air masses** form over the deserts of the southwest United States and over the deserts of Mexico. They are made of warm, dry air.

*Figure 10-1 Cloud Types*

| Cloud Name | Level | Comments |
|---|---|---|
| | Low = cloud base below 6,500 | |
| | Middle = cloud base 6,500–20,000 | |
| | High = cloud base 20,000 and up | |
| Stratus | Low | Uniform gray color. Sometimes resembles fog. |
| Altostratus | Middle | Dull gray cloud that partially obscures the sun, giving it a watery look. |
| Cirrostratus | High | These are the clouds responsible for giving the sun its halo. |
| Stratocumulus | Middle | Gray to dark gray color. Individual cells much bigger than those of altocumulus. Patches of blue sky can be seen between clouds. |
| Altocumulus | Middle | Seen in the morning, may indicate thundershowers in the afternoon. |
| Cirrocumulus | High | Small puffs high in the sky. Often develop into rippling rows. |
| Cumulonimbus | These giant clouds can start at the low levels and rise up to the troposphere (about 37,000 feet above sea level). | Towering thunderheads. Typically form over a cold front. Also form in the afternoons in Rocky Mountains and Sierra Nevada Mountains. |
| Cirrus | High | Thin and wispy. |
| Nimbostratus | Low | Low gray clouds associated with steady rain. |
| Cumulus | Low to middle | Distinctive cotton-ball shapes. Flat base. Usually lots of space between individual cumulus clouds. |

Air masses are what regulate the earth's temperature and keep the tropics from becoming unbearably hot and the poles from becoming even colder than they are. The air masses travel as warm or cold fronts thousands of miles across the oceans and continents, bringing with them changes in temperature and weather.

When a cold front meets a body of warm air, it acts as a sort of blunt wedge, forcing itself under the lighter warm air mass. If the warm air mass has moisture in it, the moisture condenses into cumuliform clouds and often heavy thundershowers. The weather that comes with a cold front is frequently violent but short-lived. Signs of an advancing cold front include cirrus, cirrostratus, and cumulonimbus clouds, surface winds out of the southwest, upper level westerly winds, and falling barometric pressure.

Warm fronts move about half the speed of cold fronts and have a shallower profile. They travel up and over colder bodies of air due to their lighter air density. As the warm, moist air rises, it cools and condenses, creating clouds and precipitation. Warm fronts often bring steady rains or snowfall,

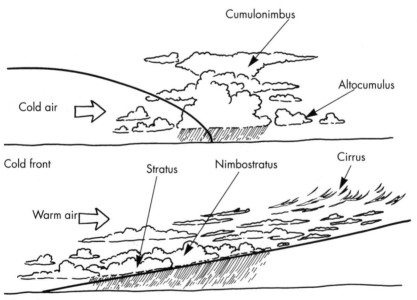

Cold fronts are characterized by their blunt wedge formation and relatively high speed of travel (about twice the speed of warm fronts). They are accompanied by cirrus, altocumulus, and cumulonimbus clouds, as well as a drop in the barometric pressure and surface winds out of the southwest.

Warm fronts don't usually bring the violent thunderstorms associated with cold fronts, but any precipitation usually lasts longer. Clouds associated with warm fronts are cirrus, stratus, and nimbostratus.

not so violent as the weather associated with cold fronts but longer lasting. The clouds that come with the approach of a warm front begin as a thin film of cirrus and cirrostratus clouds. The ice crystals in the cirrostratus clouds sometimes create a halo around the sun. As the front moves closer, the clouds thicken with the arrival of altocumulus, altostratus, and finally, nimbostratus clouds. These clouds give the sky a leaden appearance and nearly blot out the sun. The surface winds that spell the approach of a warm front blow from the southeast.

## Orographic Uplift

Certain mountain chains create their own weather with their abrupt topography. In the Sierra Nevada Mountains and in the Rocky Mountains, hikers and climbers can expect what's called orographic uplift nearly every summer day. Air moving from the west to the east hits the mountain range and is forced up thousands of feet by the topography. As the air is pushed above the mountains, it expands, cools, forms clouds, and sometimes forms violent thunderstorms. The thunderstorms usually develop in the afternoon because the heat coming off the mountains pushes the air up more violently. The clouds appear on the western horizon as innocent cumulus clouds—the fluffy cotton balls—but soon become towering cumulonimbus as they pass over the mountains. The person hiking or climbing in the Sierra Nevada Mountains or the Rockies should be aware of this "afternoon buildup" and plan accordingly. In Colorado and Wyoming, for instance, many experienced mountaineers impose a time limit on their alpine ascents so as to avoid this orographic weather. It's wise to get a very early start in the morning and summit the high peaks by early afternoon (1:00 or 2:00 P.M.) or turn back. The same goes for high passes, which are equally prone to thunderstorms.

## Lightning

Lightning strikes planet Earth about 100 times per second and kills upwards of 150 people per year in the United States. The chances of being hit by lightning are minuscule, but you certainly work the odds against yourself by standing on an exposed ridge in the middle of a violent storm. Lightning is really just a giant spark between two clouds, between a cloud and the air around it, or between a cloud and the earth. Meteorologists theorize that the motion of water and ice particles polarizes a cloud, giving it a positive charge

## Weather Tips

▾ Study the weather of the area where you'll be traveling in advance so you know the extremes and typical patterns to expect.

▾ Be prepared for the worst with sufficient clothing and good equipment.

▾ Learn the signs of approaching cold and warm fronts so you can prepare for the weather they bring.

▾ Mornings typically have more stable weather than afternoons.

on top and a negative charge on the bottom. The earth, normally a negatively charged body, develops a local positive charge from the electrostatic repulsion of the storm cloud. When the potential difference between the cloud and the earth gets strong enough (measured in millions of volts), lightning strikes. The current in a bolt of lightning reaches tens of thousands of amperes and a temperature of millions of degrees.

The heat of a lightning bolt expands and contracts the surrounding air violently, which is what causes thunder. The time, measured in seconds, between the flash of lightning and the sound of thunder gives us a good approximation of the distance between our position and the lightning strike. Every second represents about 1,100 feet. If you count to ten between the flash of lightning and the clap of thunder, followed by nine and then eight, you know the storm is moving in your direction.

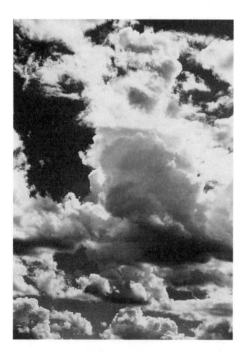

Cumulonimbus clouds. In the western mountain states, these clouds typically form during summer afternoons and sometimes bring violent thunderstorms. Cumulonimbus clouds can also signal an approaching cold front. *Theo Singelis*

## The Dos and Don'ts of Lightning

▾ Stay off high peaks and ridges. Even if you can only descend a little way off these high points, you reduce your chances of getting hit.

▾ Avoid shallow caves and overhangs. The ground current can jump gaps and electrocute the person standing in the gap.

▾ Stay away from lone trees or lone, tall objects of any sort. The tall objects are likely to get hit and, if near them, you can get hit by the ground charge.

▾ Keep your distance from metal objects and bodies of water. Both are good electrical conductors and prone to attracting lightning bolts.

▾ When possible, insulate yourself from the ground with a sleeping pad or a sleeping bag (only if you can keep it dry). Squat down with your feet close together so that in the event you do get hit by the ground charge, it travels through your feet instead of through your entire body.

▾ When traveling in a group, spread out (30 feet or more apart) so that if a party member is struck, the others can give first aid.

▾ If a person is hit by lightning and his heart stops, you have a good chance of reviving him with CPR.

▾ Avoid open spaces.

▾ In the outdoors, the best place to be in a lightning storm is in a group of trees.

Lightning is electricity and acts as such. It will follow the path of least resistance to strike the earth, and that usually means the shortest path. High points like peaks and tall trees get struck by lightning simply because they are closer to the positively charged cloud bottoms. Objects that conduct electricity well like steel posts, bodies of water, and again, trees (because of their water content) are good candidates for lightning strikes and should be avoided as well.

When lightning strikes, its electricity can travel through the ground in a broad area. This ground current is what kills most people in lightning-related accidents. Even if the tall, lone tree near you takes the full blast of the lightning bolt, you can take quite a hit just from the emanating current. For this very reason one particularly dangerous place to be in a lightning storm is in the mouth of a shallow cave. The ground current can travel to the cave's lip and jump the gap (like the spark generated by a spark plug), shocking anyone huddled there.

You may find yourself in a lightning storm someday with no forest to hide in and nothing but open space and a lone tree. Your best bet in these situations may be to crouch in "the cone of protection." The cone of protection is an imaginary circle drawn around a high point such as a lone tree or a peak. If you take a lone tree that is 100 feet tall and project a line coming at a 45-degree angle down from the top of the tree to the ground, the circumference described by that line indicates the cone of protection. The theory is that a person is safer on the edge of the cone

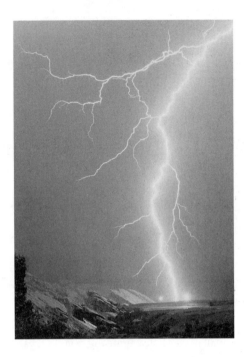

The current in a bolt of lightning reaches tens of thousands of amperes and a temperature of millions of degrees. *Ken Krehbiel*

of protection than next to the tree or out in the open far away from the tree. If everything goes according to plan, lightning will strike the tree instead of you, and you will be far enough from the base to avoid getting hit by the ground charge.

### Interview with Pamela Eaton of the Wilderness Society

Pamela Eaton is regional director of the Four Corners states for the Wilderness Society. A former NOLS instructor, Eaton has worked for the Wilderness Society for 10 years. Prior to that she earned a master's degree in natural resource policy at the University of Michigan and worked for the U.S. Park Service. According to Jerry Greenberg, director of strategic projects at the Wilderness Society, "With her background in biology and a tremendous knowledge of public policy, Pamela is one of the most effective conservationists working today."

**Q:** What keeps you optimistic about the conservation work you do?

**A:** Victories like the passage of the California Desert Protection Act. Twenty-five years ago, to even conceive of the Congress passing legislation to protect a desert landscape was laughable. The fact that Congress recently protected 7,000,000 acres of desert is reason for optimism.

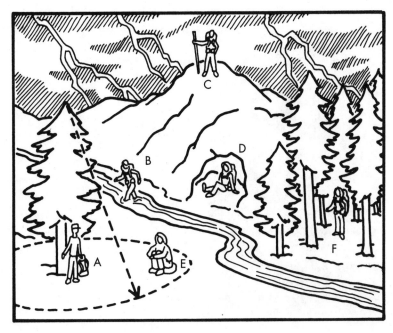

In a lightning storm, get off the high places like peaks and ridges; avoid shallow caves; avoid conductive materials like steel objects and water; and stay away from tall, lone objects. Probably the safest place to be is in a forest. If you do find yourself in the open, the "cone of protection" offers some cover. The cone of protection is a circle defined by an imaginary line extended at a 45-degree angle from the top of the tallest object in the vicinity. Inside this circle you could be struck by the ground charge of lightning that hits the tall object. Outside the cone, you may draw a direct charge yourself. Figures A, B, C, and D are the most vulnerable in this drawing. Figure F is in the safest place. Figure E sits in the "cone of protection."

**Q:** What discourages you in your work?

**A:** I try not to get discouraged but, as someone once said, in conservation work, every victory is temporary and every defeat permanent. When someone builds a logging road in a wild area there is no going back. But when we succeed in getting protective legislation passed, the Congress can always overturn it. For instance, up in the Boundary Waters, conservationists succeeded in getting Congress to pass legislation phasing out motorboats and prohibiting trucks and jeeps on portages in the wilderness. Now there are bills in the House and Senate to reopen those areas to motorized use. We are facing bills to build roads in designated wilderness in the Izembek National Wildlife Refuge in Alaska, Hells Canyon in Idaho, and in national parks. These are all places we thought were permanently protected for future generations. But rather than get discouraged, we have to renew our commitment to defend these last wild places.

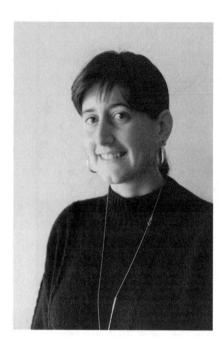

Pamela Eaton, a dedicated conservationist, works as regional director of the Four Corners states for the Wilderness Society.
*The Wilderness Society*

**Q:** How can we inspire young people to eventually get involved in land conservation?

**A:** Despite their reputation, lots of Gen-Xers see that they are facing an impoverished world and want to do something about it. I think it's important that young people see the political victories in conservation work, not just the losses. I also think it helps to introduce young people to nature no matter where you live.

   When I lived in Washington, D.C., there was this little swamp called Huntley Meadows. It is surrounded by urban sprawl. Whenever I went there, I noticed that it was the children who stopped to look at the creepy crawly things—crayfish and spiders and things like that. The adults noticed the bigger, obvious animals like the birds, but it was the children who stopped the adults to look at the little things. I think children reawaken the awe for nature in adults.

**Q:** Who are your heroes in the conservation world?

**A:** My heroes are some of the very people who started the Wilderness Society: Aldo Leopold, Bob Marshall, and Howard Zahnhiser, who wrote the Wilderness Act. They had a vision of the American landscape and saw themselves as being able to change how civilization treated the lands. They were successful in that. Part of what motivates me working here at the Wilderness Society is knowing I'm carrying on that legacy.

   Terry Tempest Williams is also a hero of mine because she communicates her passion for the land, and her writing helps renew my spirits and passion for nature.

**Q:** What advice would you have for someone who wants to get involved in conservation work?

**A:** You have to ask yourself how you can be most effective. For some people that means sitting in a tree that's about to be chopped down. For others, it means testifying before Congress. Sitting in a tree isn't for everyone and testifying before Congress isn't for everyone either, so you have to find your own way to make the world a more friendly place for nature. Even just writing a letter helps. There's a whole spectrum of opinions out there from the most passionate advocates to the most passionate opponents. It's not always easy to be a passionate defender of the land. There are times when people disagree. That's healthy—that's democracy.

You have to renew your awe for nature from time to time. As we become adults we can lose our passion for nature beneath all our rational thinking. It's the awe that people feel that makes conservation work happen.

# CHAPTER 11

# Cooking in the Backcountry

'Tis an ill cook that cannot lick his own fingers.

—William Shakespeare, *Romeo and Juliet*, act 4, scene 2

While the rest of the world boiled their freeze-dried turkey tetrazzini, nursed their high-altitude headaches, and melted chunks of the glacier for their miserable herbal tea at the camp 15,000 feet up Denali, my climbing partner Lannie Hamilton fashioned a pizza. With no firewood, water melted from snow, and sauce from tomato powder, she made us a pizza that had a fluffy golden crust, structural integrity, and, most important, was very good to the palate. I can report to you that it was one of the best pizzas I have ever had and certainly was the best pizza on Denali that day in May. But don't take my word for it, take the word of the Japanese team camped next to us. Moments after Lannie finished baking, the Japanese were making trading gestures—their dried fish for a slice of our pizza. With the trading skills that have made the Japanese an economic powerhouse, they swapped six dried fish sticks for half of Lannie's masterpiece, and we found ourselves gnawing on something up from the Sea of Amakusa while they ate pizza and made cooing noises.

The point is, you can cook a good meal in nearly any condition in the backcountry. You can make bread, cake, pies, curry dishes, Mexican chilis, quiches, soups, stir-fries, casseroles, and almost whatever else you fancy.

Some people suspend the pleasures of the palate while on a camping trip and treat their meals in the wilderness as mere units of energy or fuel rods.

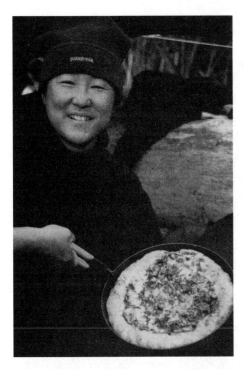

Who says you have to eat gruel on a backcountry trip? Don't cheat your inner epicure just because you're camping. A student shows off a pizza cooked on a small camp stove. *Deborah Sussex*

They bring and eat the sorts of things you might expect to find a peacekeeping unit eating while on patrol in some shaky part of the world. Typically they are easy to prepare, nutritionally balanced, loaded with energy, and taste like nuclear fuel rods. But why? The outdoors should bring out the best in your meals. You have appetite on your side. Schedule 15 miles and a 3,000-foot pass on your day to cook and, by God, your friends will rave about whatever creation you hatch from the pan that evening. You also have time in the outdoors to enjoy your meals. In the mountains, we have fewer distractions and certainly nothing distracts us from the meal at hand when we are hungry. There are few things in life more sublime than sitting down with your friends for dinner at a beautiful kitchen site when you're tired and hungry. When someone takes the trouble to cook something with a bit of skill and delicacy, what was once merely routine becomes exalted. Finally, the beautiful surroundings enhance any meal; there's no such thing as a bad table when camping. With some planning, some practice, and some imagination, you can eat well, stay within pack weight limits, and dine with a bit of style.

# Your Kitchen Site

Your kitchen should not be by your tent unless you find a particularly tough surface there. By moving your kitchen away from your tent, you distribute the trampling impact over two sites instead of concentrating it all on one site.

The best kitchen sites are protected from the wind. When there are strong winds and poor shelter, your water literally will not boil, watched or not.

Finally, look for a kitchen area that offers the best views and early morning sun (open to the east) to warm you up and inspire you. What's nicer than a cup of coffee in the early morning when you've chosen a kitchen with a superior view of a canyon or a mountain range?

# Kitchen Gear

The typical kitchen outfit includes a large pot, a frying pan, some pot grips, a large spoon, a spatula, and a water container (to get water for camp). If you are traveling alone or with one other person, you can get away with a two-quart pot. If you are traveling in a group of three or more, you should have at least a four-quart pot. Particularly with a group of three or more, consider bringing two pots. Two pots will give you the flexibility to cook one dish while preparing, say, bread dough, or heating water while mixing the pasta sauce. If you have to melt snow for your water, two pots are especially useful. A frying pan is optional and can be left behind if you need to shed weight. But for baking, frying fish, or making pancakes, you need a sturdy non-stick pan with no plastic parts (so nothing melts over a campfire).

Some people bring a small pressure cooker to save fuel and time when cooking things like beans and lentils. At very high altitudes, a pressure cooker allows you to bring your water and meals up to a much higher temperature than you could with just an aluminum pot.

# Water Treatment*

Unfortunately even the crystal-clear waters you find in the wilderness are swimming with evil bacteria, protozoa, viruses, and sometimes chemicals.

*For a good treatment of water filters and water-borne microorganisms, see the December 1996 issue of *Backpacker* magazine.

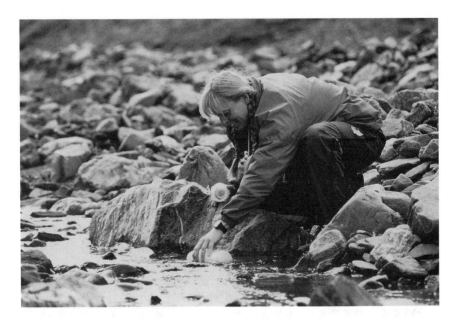

Even the crystal-clear waters in the high mountains can be contaminated with protozoa, bacteria, and viruses. To be safe, treat your water chemically or with a good filter.
*Tom Bol*

Unless proven otherwise, assume that the water you find on your trip is contaminated and filter it, treat it, or purify it.

Water should be treated either with a filter, chemically, or through heat. Today's water filters have elements that strain microorganisms as small as .2 microns. They catch protozoa and bacteria, but not viruses, which are as small as .004 microns. Some water purifiers have an iodine element to kill viruses as well. Water filters (the ones without the iodine purifier) are nice because you get good water quickly and without the chemical taste. But filters don't come cheaply. Expect to pay between $50 and $500. What do you get for more money? You get a device that cleans water faster (up to four quarts per minute), cleans more water per replacement element, filters smaller organisms, and is more durable. If you buy a water filter, study the specifications including pumping capacity in quarts per minute, lifetime (in quarts) of the filter element, and the type of microorganisms the filter will catch.

If you don't want to take a filter, you can treat your water with halogens such as iodine. Iodine is an inexpensive, effective treatment that takes care of bacteria, viruses, and protozoa except for Cryptosporidium. You can buy iodine tablets such as Potable Aqua in small bottles of 50 tablets. One tablet purifies one quart of water, though two should be used in very murky water. Allow at least 15 minutes for the tablet to dissolve before drinking it and before adding fruit crystals (the crystals can interfere with the chemical action). In very cold water, allow 45 minutes for the tablets to kill all the microorganisms. Let a little of the treated water spill onto the threads and cap of your bottle to purify them.

In a pinch, a solution of 10% povidone iodine can be used to purify water. Use 5 to 10 drops of the 2% solution per quart depending on the water's murkiness.

Boiling water kills microorganisms that commonly cause diarrhea and if your filter gets clogged or you run out of tablets, it may be your only option. You only need to bring the water to a boil to kill the microorganisms. Don't waste time and fuel keeping the water boiling an extra 10 or 20 minutes.

If you're using water in your cooking—whether for soup or for pancake batter—you needn't treat the water beforehand, as the heat from the cooking itself will do the trick.

## MICROORGANISMS IN YOUR WATER BOTTLE

Here is a list of what might be swimming in even the clearest-looking streams:

- ▼ Protozoa. Protozoa are single-cell creatures and the largest of the waterborne microorganisms. They range in size from 2 to 15 microns (about one-one-hundredth the diameter of a human hair) and can only be seen through a microscope. The most common and bothersome protozoan is Giardia lamblia, which measures from 8 to 12 microns but, because they are flexible, can fit through holes as small as 5 microns. Giardia is spread through fecal and oral transmission. In short, when Giardia-carrying mammals defecate in the water, they infect the water. Beavers and muskrats are the most likely mammals to spread Giardia, simply because they live aqueous lives. But livestock, dogs, and humans can also contaminate the water with Giardia. It only takes one Giardia cyst to infect you. Once infected, Giardia symptoms include diarrhea, flatulence, abdominal cramps, fatigue, and weight loss. The symptoms come one to four weeks after exposure.

    Another nasty protozoan, and something we've only recently become aware of, is Cryptosporidium. Cryptosporidia are smaller and more elusive than their Giardia cousins. They measure in size from 4 to 6 microns but can pinch through a 3-micron hole. What's more, they are tougher than Giardia (due to a harder shell) and won't give in to iodine or bleach. To eliminate Cryptosporidium you need to either boil your water or use a fine water filter (smaller than 3 microns). Symptoms of Cryptosporidiosis mimic Giardiasis but with less flatulence. In addition, Cryptosporidiosis victims usually have a low-grade fever.

▾ Bacteria. Bacteria are smaller than protozoa, ranging in size from .2 to 10 microns. Water-borne bacteria include cholera, Escherichia coli, and campylobacter. While there isn't much cholera in the United States, it's common in the water of certain developing countries. E-coli is found in water contaminated by feces and is one of the causes of "traveler's diarrhea."

▾ Viruses are the smallest of the microorganisms and can't be filtered. They must be boiled or chemically treated to die. A person traveling in less developed parts of the world should be aware of hepatitis A, a food- and water-borne virus that causes fatigue, nausea, stomach pain, and loss of appetite.

## Sanitation in the Kitchen

Recently I had the misfortune to go camping with a friend who had a bad cold, a runny nose, and the unpleasant habit of wiping his schnozzle with the back of his hand. I watched with fear and loathing as he sneezed, wiped his nose, and scooped me a ladle of soup, all in one smooth motion. I ate the soup with dread and sure enough, a day later I had his cold and a ruined weekend. Watching someone with filthy hands or an undressed, infected wound—someone who is hygienically challenged—cook your dinner is unsavory to say the least. Worse, their poor hygiene may make for a nauseating trip—literally.

When people imagine injuries and illnesses in the outdoors, they picture something like a sprained ankle or hypothermia. Few imagine that poor hygiene in the kitchen, or otherwise, seriously threatens their health while camping. But there are lots of underhanded germs out there in the dirt, in your food, and on your person that are just waiting for you to drop your defenses. For example, over 50 percent of the human population carries the staphylococcus aureus bacterium, a bug that can make you so ill you'll do what the medical people so delicately call "projectile vomiting."

Just six bacteria are responsible for over 90 percent of food-borne illnesses.

Bacteria grow best in an environment where the temperature is between 40 degrees and 140 degrees F. So unless you are cooking your food or camping in cold conditions, your food makes an attractive environment for bacterial growth. The safest meal is a meal that has been freshly cooked. It's best

## Sanitation Tips for the Kitchen

▼ Wash your hands thoroughly before cooking. Hands are the biggest points of communication for disease.

▼ Don't share utensils, water bottles, lip balm, etc. If you want to share water, pour it into your friend's cup or bottle.

▼ Don't use personal utensils to cook with. Don't eat from group utensils such as the cooking spoon. If you need to taste the dish you're cooking, use the group spoon to move food to your own bowl.

▼ Avoid leftovers. A pot of food stored between 40° and 140° F makes the perfect environment for bacterial growth.

▼ Wash your dishes thoroughly and sanitize them with either hot water or a chlorine-treated wash.

to avoid leftovers. If you cook a big pot of macaroni and cheese, eat half and then leave half for the morning, your pot has the potential to become a bacteria colony overnight.

You get dirty camping and hiking all day and it's not easy to keep everything clean. But taking the time to wash your dishes well, wash your hands before cooking, not eating from the pot with your spoon, and not sharing each other's water bottles and lip balm certainly reduces the risk of getting a gastrointestinal illness. Taking this little bit of trouble to be hygienic in the outdoors goes even further in large groups of people.

# Basic Cooking in the Backcountry

One of the secrets to cooking well in the backcountry is to spend a little time setting up your kitchen nicely and organizing everything you need to prepare your meal before you even light the stove. If your kitchen site is dry, sheltered, comfortable, and has a bit of flat space to organize your food and position your stove, you will be infinitely more efficient than you would with a precarious site and no space. If you organize your utensils, the ingredients of the meal, and keep some fashion of organization throughout the cooking process, chances are your meal will come out better: You'll be less likely to forget an important spice, overcook a dish while you fish around for an ingredient, or lose a utensil in the grass.

Nylon zip bags are very helpful to keep you organized. On long trips, if you have two or three zip bags, you would do well to get in the habit of compartmentalizing them. You might use one for breakfast and trail foods, and the other for dinners, desserts, and spices. On longer trips you will also generate a substantial amount of garbage—food scraps, leftovers, plastic bags, etc. Use plastic bags (doubled) to keep your garbage safely in one place. Work on consolidating like ingredients as you go through your ration. No sense

*Figure 11-1 The Six Most Common Food-Borne Illnesses*

| Name | Where Found | Time From Ingestion to Illness | Symptoms |
| --- | --- | --- | --- |
| Clostridium perfingens | On meat stored in a too-warm environment | 8–24 hours | Nausea, diarrhea, abdominal cramps |
| Campylobacter jejuni | Meats, water sources, feces | 4–7 days | Stomach pain, bloody diarrhea |
| Bacillus cereus | Grains and spices | 8–16 hours | Stomach pain, nausea, vomiting, diarrhea |
| Shigella | Food and water contaminated by fecal matter | 3–7 days | Bloody, mucus-ridden diarrhea |
| Staphylococcus aureus | Protein rich foods stored at warm temperatures | 30 minutes–6 hours | Cramps, vomiting, diarrhea, headaches, sweats, and chills |
| Salmonella | Eggs, dairy products | 12–24 hours | Stomach pain, diarrhea, nausea, vomiting, headache, chills, weakness, thirst |

having four or five small bags of milk powder scattered throughout your ration when one will do.

Everyone has certain likes and dislikes when it comes to food and there's no accounting for taste. Consider that some people like haggis, the Scottish dish of minced heart, lungs, and liver all mixed with oatmeal. Pray you never camp with them, but try to accommodate and respect their tastes if you do. It's always a challenge to keep everyone happy when all you have is one aluminum pot and ingredients from your pack to cook with. The point is to find out what people like and don't like and then strike a happy medium in your camp meals. I happen to like nearly all my food spiced to nuclear levels, but it's not fair for me to splash cayenne over every meal I cook if my camp partner was raised on cabbage and boiled beef. If there are disparities in taste, you can cook a very basic—read nonspiced—dish and each person can spice his or her dish.

## BAKING

When I took my first NOLS course, my instructor astounded us by baking a loaf of bread on a tiny camping stove. He did all the normal things one does to bake bread—activating yeast, kneading the dough, letting it rise, and then finally baking it. But the fact that he could create a feathery loaf of bread on some godforsaken beach out in the middle of Mexico with just one small camp stove and some finesse with a twiggy fire caused us students to address him with a certain amount of veneration the rest of the trip. But baking in the backcountry—while it takes a little practice—just isn't that hard to do. And if you know how to bake on a camp stove or over the coals of a fire, you can add so much to your backcountry menu with breads, pizzas, cinnamon rolls, and desserts. One of the nicest touches to a breakfast on a rest day is freshly baked cinnamon rolls; calzones or the like make your dinners much more fun.

The best days to bake are the warm days when you have extra time in the morning or the evening. Even if you've never baked bread, don't be intimidated by yeast. Granted, there are times when the yeast won't activate—whether from the cold, too hot water, or just plain bad yeast—but with a little practice you'll find baking with yeast to be a simple task.

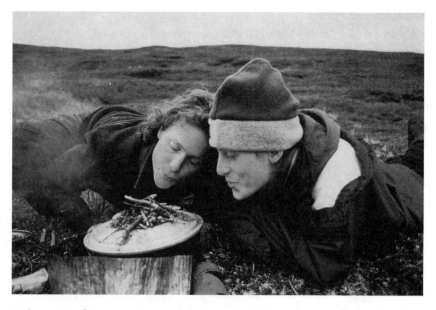

With a twiggy fire, a camp stove, and some imagination, you can bake anything from bread to coffee cake. *Frederik Norrsell*

## Baking Tips

▼ Your dough will expand as you bake it, so don't fill the pan more than about half full with dough.

▼ If you are above treeline or an area where there is little or no wood, you can flip the pan to bake each side. Start with an extra-stiff dough.

▼ On cold days or cold nights, put your rising dough in a plastic bag and keep it inside your sleeping bag or against your chest to keep it warm.

▼ Add variety to your breads by adding spices such as basil and oregano, cheese, and rehydrated vegetables such as peppers, tomatoes, and onions.

The first thing you need to do is to activate the yeast with warm water and a couple of tablespoons of sugar. Warm the water to the point where it feels warm on your wrist but does not burn your skin—about the temperature of a very warm bath. A large insulated mug is a good place to activate your yeast because it will keep the water warm. Fill your mug about two-thirds full with the warm water (about 1½ cups), add two tablespoons of sugar (to feed the yeast), a couple of teaspoons of salt (for flavor), and then a tablespoon of yeast. Let the mixture stand in a warm place for about ten minutes. By then you should have a good head of foam from the activated yeast. If you do not see at least a quarter inch of foam after ten minutes, the yeast hasn't activated properly—either from too warm water, too cold water, or too old yeast—and you'll have to try again with a totally new batch.

Pour the yeast water in the biggest pot you have and add half the flour. Stir the mix vigorously for about three minutes. Gradually add the remaining flour, mixing with a spoon. Keep adding flour until you have a springy dough that won't stick to your hands. Now flour your hands and knead the dough vigorously (the inside of a clean frying pan makes a good surface) for about ten minutes. If the dough is sticky, add more flour. Ultimately you want your dough to be springy to the touch.

Once kneaded, the dough needs time to rise in a warm setting. If it's the middle of summer on a warm day, you can leave the dough in a covered pot and let it sit in the sun for an hour. Be sure to oil the pot first and put a little oil on top of your dough, too. On the bitter cold days, I have seen NOLS instructors, desperate for something baked, sleep with a rising dough or keep it in a plastic bag against their chest, with good results.

After the dough has risen about an hour, knead it again about ten minutes. If you have the time and can let the dough rise a second time, you will get a fluffier bread. If you don't have the time, you can bake it after just one rising.

Oil a frying pan (margarine works too) and shape the dough to fit the inside of the pan. The best way to bake the dough is to make a Dutch oven out of your frying pan and frying pan lid. You can use your stove turned on a very low heat for the lower source of heat and build a "twiggy" fire on the lid of your frying pan. Make your twiggy fire out of branches no bigger than the diameter of a quarter. Your fire should be hot, but not so hot that you burn your hand when it's held six to eight inches from the lid. Since your stove is too small to heat up the entire bottom of the frying pan, you need to rotate the pan over the stove so the entire bottom gets cooked evenly, also known as "baking around the clock." Place the pan on the stove off-center and then every few minutes rotate the pan about a third turn.

Baking bread over a camp stove takes anywhere from about 30 to 50 minutes. The bread is done when it makes a hollow thumping noise when tapped with a spoon.

## BOILING

Staple foods like rice, pasta, and soups really need only boiling to cook. Nevertheless, there are a few things you should know about boiling in the backcountry. I have mentioned this before, but it's worth mentioning again: An unprotected pot of water sitting on a camp stove in a strong wind will take eons to reach a boil, and, if the wind is strong and cold enough, the pot just won't boil. So, do everything you can to shelter your pot. Pick a natural alcove for your stove, use the windscreen provided by the stove manufacturer, and surround the stove and pot with rocks or food bags. Most importantly, use your pot lid.

If you're cooking pasta, be sure to bring the water to a full boil before tossing in the noodles. Even at sea level, pasta becomes gluey when put in less than boiling water. At high altitudes, where water boils at a lower temperature, it's even more important to wait for the full boil before throwing in the pasta.

With rice, the reverse is true. It's best to put rice in a pot of cold water and then bring it to a boil. I have also heard it said that rice cooks better if you don't stir it and don't remove the pot's lid until you think the rice is done. Stirring the rice too much will make it starchy and gluey.

If you want soup with your meal on nights when you make pasta, you can use the hot water from your pasta to make your soup. It saves time and fuel.

## FRYING

If you bring a frying pan on your trip, you can fry trout, pasta, rice, hash browns, and even bread dough. Fried foods have lots of flavor and lots of fat

## Cooking Tips from Sam Talucci

Sam Talucci is a NOLS instructor and restaurateur of some 20 years. A gourmet in the woods and at home in Philadelphia, Sam would sooner ditch his tent than even the lowliest spice. Here are some of Sam's cooking tips for the outdoors:

▼ Consider bringing olive oil instead of margarine. It's healthier and tastes better. Replace a pound of margarine with about 16 oz. of oil.

▼ If you catch trout, try dredging them in cornmeal and then sprinkle with a mix of Coleman's mustard, dill, and Spike. Fry in margarine or olive oil.

▼ Sun-dried tomatoes and dried shiitake mushrooms are great extras to bring. They make a big addition to dishes like risotto or backcountry pizza. Dried cherries are hard to find, but they make a great addition to any cobbler.

▼ If you want to add a little gourmet to your life, bring a small air-dried salami (it keeps well) and serve it with black pepper biscuits and some Coleman's mustard.

▼ Dressing for backcountry greens: olive oil, vinegar, soy, mustard, Spike, and dill. (You can also add a little curry to this dressing.)

▼ When frying foods, especially if you're doing several things in the kitchen at once, add a little water to the pan. It helps to keep things from sticking to the pan and you can still get that nice golden look.

▼ For fried dishes such as fried rice or risotto, fry the spices in a little olive oil first. It brings out the flavors.

(good for energy). Fried pasta is a nice variation from the usual. Boil your pasta as you normally would and then fry it in oil or margarine and spices such as oregano, garlic, rehydrated onion flakes, salt and pepper. You can do the same with rice dishes. Cook your rice in water as you normally would and then fry it for a nice texture and flavor.

Some NOLS instructors hold a certain reverence for the whole act of frying foods and especially for those who do it well. They speak of the "courage to fry," and the three attending forms of courage that go with it:

▼ The courage to use lots of grease
▼ The courage to burn
▼ The courage not to stir the pan too often

What they're getting at is that fried dishes work best if you turn up the heat and then really fry your food with plenty of oil or margarine, without fussing around too much with your spatula. I suppose it does take a certain odd form of courage to do it right.

One way to bring out the flavor in your fried dishes is to fry your spices in a little oil first.

## Cooking in Your Tent

Cooking in your tent is usually not a good idea for a few reasons. First of all, even the best camp stoves emit toxic fumes that will poison your brain with carbon monoxide if they become trapped in your tent. Some campers have died from carbon monoxide poisoning while cooking in their tent. Second, tents are made of flammable materials that will go up in a hurry if a stove falls over or if you have a fuel leak.

## Cleaning Up

Get in the habit of cleaning up your kitchen every night before you go to bed so animals don't ransack your food supplies, you can find things in the morning when it's time to cook breakfast, and so your dishes don't turn into petri dishes. You've already been warned of the nasty bacteria inhabiting the microworlds of your food, so washing dishes bears a mention. Some people like to bring a small abrasive pad on their trips to wash dishes. On short trips that works fine, but on longer trips the thing usually becomes an ungodly mess of food scraps and bacteria. Plain sand or mineral soil seems to be about the best thing for scouring dishes. Things like pine cones and pine boughs work well too. Wash your dishes well away from water sources so you don't contaminate them. Providing you have enough fuel, give your dishes a hot rinse every day or two to sterilize them.

## Dehydrating Your Own Food

Some of my favorite foods out in the mountains are fruits, vegetables, and meats that I've dehydrated myself. Home-dehydrated food is intensely flavorful, lightweight, inexpensive, and can make your menu much more interesting. You can dehydrate food in an oven or even in the sun, but commercial food dehydrators are inexpensive ($100 to $150) and easier to use. You can dehydrate tomatoes, for instance, then rehydrate them in the field to use with your spaghetti sauce or pizza. Dehydrate peppers or jalapeños and add some fire to your dinners. Dehydrating is easy to do and requires only slicing, blanching, and drying.

Another option is to make your own fruit leathers, which make easy trail snacks. Fruit leathers are simple to make: Just wash the raw fruit of your choice, puree in a blender (with a little sugar if you like), pour the puree onto plastic wrap on the shelf of your dehydrator, and then dry for 6 to 8 hours per side. A variation is to cook the fruit first, force it through a sieve or colander, and then dehydrate as described above.

I love jerky, but find most of the commercial types too expensive and too loaded with long and ponderous ingredients to be much fun. It's not difficult to make your own jerky and out in the wilderness it's a great source of protein. Here's a simple recipe I use with game and beef.

*2–3 pounds of meat (The best cuts are the low-fat ones like round and flank steak.)*

*Marinade:*
*1 cup soy sauce*
*1 cup Worcestershire sauce*
*Juice of 1 lemon*
*1 tablespoon fresh ground pepper*
*2–3 cloves chopped garlic*
*½ onion, chopped*
*1 teaspoon Tabasco sauce (optional)*

1. Slice the meat into strips about ¼ to ⅜ inch thick and 1½ inches wide. It's easiest to slice the meat if it's partially frozen.
2. Trim off the fat (the fat does not keep as well as the rest of the meat and may cause your jerky to spoil).
3. Put the meat in a ceramic, glass, or plastic bowl (metal bowls react with the ingredients) and cover with the marinade.
4. Marinate meat between 6 and 12 hours.
5. Drain off marinade and place strips of meat on oven rack or dehydrator.
6. Dehydrate about 4–6 hours per side in open-doored oven or dehydrator set at about 140 degrees.

**Note:** Dehydrating times can vary considerably depending on the oven or the dryer. Some meat will dry faster than other meat, depending on its thickness and position in the oven or dryer. Once dried, jerky should be leathery but not brittle. Experiment with times until you get the texture you like. Jerky is best stored in zip-lock bags in the refrigerator. Out on the trail, it will last several weeks.

# Natural Additions

Living entirely off the land without rations is difficult, and you must know how to scavenge to keep yourself fed. But nearly everywhere you go you can find something growing near your campsite or along the trail to add to your meals. Do keep in mind that there are some poisonous plants out there too: To the untrained eye, the toxic water hemlock looks much like the edible cow parsnip. The death camus looks like certain wild onions. Mushrooms are especially tricky. While there are certain edible mushrooms that are unmistakable, others are not so obvious. The point is, you should educate yourself with a good field guide and some advice from an experienced naturalist.

Trout are always a nice addition to any meal. You can dredge them in cornmeal or flour and salt and pepper and then fry them in oil or margarine. You can also add trout to rice dishes, soups, and casseroles.

Keep your eyes open for edible greens. You can make backcountry salads from bluebells, miner's leaf, spring beauties, dandelions, and mountain sorrel. If you remembered to bring oil and vinegar, you can make a dressing and truly dine in style. Early in the season, elk thistle makes a nice celery-like appetizer. Nettles make excellent soup and are said to have medicinal qualities as well. Some regions have wild onions. As it gets later in the season, the mountain berries ripen and, with a bit of foraging, you can gather enough strawberries, raspberries, serviceberries, chokecherries, or buffalo berries to add to your pancakes or cobbler. Mushrooms and puffballs come out late in the summer too. Wild mushrooms sautéed in butter are exquisite. Wild mushrooms on your pizza or as an addition to a pasta dish—words escape me here. But until you have truly learned to distinguish edible mushrooms from the poisonous ones, don't take any chances here.

## Food Stress

The darker side of dining comes with real or imagined scarcity. Some people, usually novice campers, worry that they'll not get enough to eat and food becomes an exaggerated point of focus. They might monitor what everyone in the group eats down to the individual peanut or spoon of oatmeal. Worse, they might make clandestine forays into the food and eat much more than the allotted ration. In such cases, food brings out the worst in people— hoarding, selfishness, and pettiness. When food is truly scarce on a trip, you may really need to carefully ration what little you have. But if you have planned your ration correctly and not incurred huge delays on your trip, you and your tentmates should have plenty to eat.

# CHAPTER 12

# Our Responsibility to the Land

Something will have gone out of us as a people if we ever let the remaining wilderness be destroyed; if we permit the last virgin forests to be turned into comic books and plastic cigarette cases . . . We simply need that wild country available to us, even if we never do more than drive to its edge and look in. For it can be a means of reassuring ourselves of our sanity as creatures, a part of the geography of hope.

—Wallace Stegner, *Wilderness Letter*

A rancher friend of mine by the name of Max is having problems with the elk. They're eating all his hay before he gets a chance to cut it. In June and July, when his alfalfa and oats are rich and green, 100 or so elk move onto his fields and gorge themselves.

"They love that alfalfa," Max says. "It's like a drug for them."

June and July is an odd time for this elk herd to be down at such a low altitude—about 6,500 feet. Historically the elk of western Colorado have ranged the high country above 8,000 feet in the summer.

But the high country has become a busy place with all the recreationists on off-road vehicles (ORVs), and the elk feel safer down low on Max's land, where there's just one rancher armed with an irrigation shovel and some awfully well-grown alfalfa.

Max has nothing against elk. Ten years ago, when the elk still spent summers in the high country, he hardly gave them a thought. Today, however, they're eating into his profits—literally—and threatening his way of life.

Max has asked the state wildlife agents for payment to compensate him for his losses, but they won't give it to him. And the elk won't be chased off his land either.

Where would they go? Lower down, the valley has a major highway running through it, subdivisions of suburban housing, and a golf course. The elk go to the golf course too, but the club has the manpower and a fleet of golf carts to chase them off.

So the elk go to Max's place and are happy there for the moment. But the situation can't last. The profit margins in ranching are thin to begin with; a stretch of land can only support so many animals and produce so much hay.

Down the road, the elk herd will have to be reduced, ORV traffic in the high country will have to be restricted, or Max will have to find another way to make a living.

The plight of Max and his alfalfa is but one small example of what's happening everywhere in this country and beyond: Humans and wildlife are having a hard time finding enough space to live together. It's no wonder. In the last 70 years, since the U.S. government first did an inventory, the number of roadless areas—or wildlife habitat—has probably been quartered (the exact number of roadless areas is a matter of dispute today).

In Africa, some 12,000 miles east of Max's ranch, Kenyan farmers are having the same sort of problem as Max, but with animals a little higher on the food chain: lions. An article in the August 12, 1998, issue of the New York Times tells one such story. In the small town of Kitengala, lions have killed more than 20 cattle in the last two months, and one farmer lost 10 goats and sheep in one night to the big cats. In 1946, Kenya had 5,000,000 people; today it has upwards of 30,000,000 people. The consequences of more people on a fixed amount of arable land are obvious. The once wild savannas around the national parks are being farmed and bringing people into rangelands that once belonged exclusively to the animals. Just as the elk find Max's alfalfa irresistible, the lions can't resist a fat steer or ewe.

The contest between mankind and the wilds has a history of thousands if not millions of years. But not long ago, the sides were more evenly matched. It used to be that we had crude tools to do our hunting and farming. Maybe back then surviving did mean a battle against nature. Today we have such good machines and systems of production that the preservation or the breaking of the wilds is entirely a choice to be made by humankind.

Some would argue that the effort to save the wild places is not worth it— that we would be better off if we farmed and factoried every square foot, save for a little land to build fairways for Sunday golf. Left to men like Robert Moses, who built New York State's major highways and parkways and once said, "A lot of people . . . hate the country and love congestion," we probably wouldn't have many places left to go canoeing, backpacking, climbing, or birdwatching.

But we are not purely creatures of utility. Nearly since our founding as a nation we have had strong voices in support of wilderness. Who knows exactly when it began? Perhaps, as many writers have suggested, it started with James Fenimore Cooper and his fictional character Natty Bumppo, or "Leatherstocking." While the rest of the country raced to fell and mill every tree from Maine to what is now Oregon, to plow every level acre, and to graze every blade of grass, Cooper's Leatherstockings thrived in the wilds and mourned its domestication.

Since Cooper we have had Henry David Thoreau, Ralph Waldo Emerson, John Muir, Theodore Roosevelt, Olaus and Margaret Murie, Justice William O. Douglas, Rosalie Edge, Rachel Carson, Harold Ickes, John D. Rockefeller, David Brower, Edward Abbey, and Terry Tempest Williams. All of them spoke and acted forcefully for the cultural, aesthetic, and spiritual value of the "untrammeled."

The conservation ethic comes from the belief that the good life means more than what we can extract from the land. It comes from the conviction that wilderness helps us keep our sanity, our hope, and our humility. This last trait, humility, is part and parcel of the conservation ethic. For the ethic lives and breathes in the people who believe that our species—the fortunate ones with the biggest brains and the opposable thumbs—don't own the world outright. Just because we have it within our means to appropriate every square inch of the earth and decide which species may live and which are too much of a nuisance doesn't mean we should. As Aldo Leopold put it, ". . . a land ethic

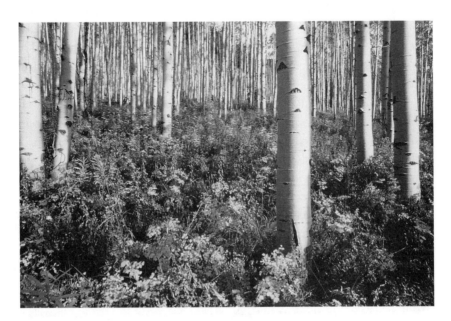

An aspen forest protected by a conservation act. *Mark Harvey*

changes the role of Homo sapiens from conqueror of the land-community to plain member and citizen of it. It implies respect for his fellow members, and also respect for the community as such."*

It takes a leap in logic to include the small biota—the spiders, voles, plainest of birds, even the fungi—on our list of worthwhile life forms. And it takes a nearly biblical world view to defend their right to live on the planet despite their apparent lack of cash value, stunning beauty, or charisma. But let's just say for a moment that we are purely creatures of utility and our species is the only one that matters. Given that self-importance, do we really know how to manage a planet several billion years in the making? Are we quite so confident that we can headlong change the soils, oceans, and atmosphere to produce our worldly goods and comforts? Might there be something integral to the complexities of the biota—the biodiversity—that sustains our species? The idea that the entire world—the water, prairies, forests, desert, and mountains—is meant only to be fodder for the human trough is a conceit and hubris that would leave us poorer if not in real trouble.

The land ethic is alive in this country. I have the pleasure of serving as a board member on a small nonprofit foundation aimed at funding groups and individuals who fight the good fight to protect the wild places and the animals who live there. We meet but once a year to review grant proposals and I am always heartened reading them. It's encouraging to see the dozens of small groups seeking $5,000 or so to fight a legal battle against some behemoth mining company or timber conglomerate, where $5,000 would be lost on the balance sheet. Here's a request for $2,000 to do some of the spadework for reintroducing grizzly bears to Colorado (the last one was killed in 1979). The group has some hard work ahead and some strong odds against success: Colorado has a law on its books prohibiting the reintroduction of the grizzly and the wolf. Here's a group requesting $3,000 to protect wetlands in Idaho and Wyoming, home to great gray owls, whooping cranes, neotropical passerines, and others. But the county where they hope to protect these wetlands is growing at a rate of 10 percent, the sixth fastest in the United States. It goes without saying that this group will meet fierce adversaries in the real estate companies and developers who have one-eighth-acre parcels and commissions on the mind.

Most of these environmental groups are small, scrappy organizations that get through the year on paltry budgets, volunteer labor, and the conviction that saving some habitat, wilderness, clean water—saving the untamed and unbroken parts of the world—is worth their time and considerable efforts.

*Aldo Leopold, *A Sand County Almanac*, Oxford University Press, 1989, p. 204.

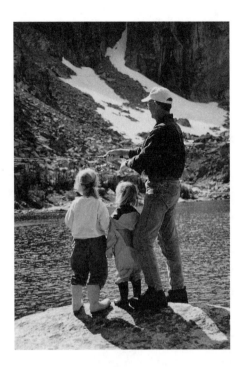

Marshall and Catherine Brame fishing with Jack Chadwick in the Wind River Mountains. *Rich Brame*

It's not that the conservation ethic doesn't exist, it's that there are tremendous economic, political, and social forces working against conservation. We have a great history of conservation in the United States matched only by a great history of ravaging the nicer places. The drive to preserve wilderness areas, habitat, and other species has run a parallel course with the economic forces that see only the stock in trade and utility of an area. The battle is sure to grow fiercer over the next 50 years as we add another two to four billion people to the world and once-subsistent economies try to advance their standard of living to the level of "first world." If it's hard to keep oil corporations from getting their mitts on Alaska's delicate north today, imagine the pressures 20 years from now when today's developed oilfields run dry. Certainly the only thing that will keep a few corners of the earth wild is a voting, letter-writing, protesting, fund-raising public.

You may be wondering what all this has to do with you, just a guy or gal who wanted to go backpacking and bought this book to learn how to use a compass or plan a trip. But trust me here, the land ethic and your trip to the backcountry are related. When you pitch your tent on a rock shelf instead of over a bed of broad-leafed shoots you have preserved a small square of wilderness. When you build just a small fire with dead and downed wood (or no fire at all), you leave a place in better condition than does the fellow who builds a raging bonfire and strips the branches of nearby trees. To camp well

## Five Things You Can Do to Make a Difference

▾ Inform yourself on an issue. Read books, magazines, newspapers, visit Web pages, and watch television shows that keep you abreast of the most important conservation issues.

▾ Write a letter to the city council, a congressman, a land manager, or to the newspaper. A well-written letter that outlines the facts and your beliefs on an issue can sway the opinion of those who make decisions. A letter published in a newspaper or magazine can inform others on an issue and stir up action among those who share your beliefs.

▾ Go to public hearings and speak out. Many government bodies are required by law to hold public hearings on land-use decisions. Just one person who speaks his or her opinion can make a big difference.

▾ Join a group. There are hundreds (if not thousands) of local, national, and international groups that do good conservation work. These groups lobby lawmakers, buy land for protection, fund studies, and educate the public. Your membership usually gets you a newsletter subscription and your fees help keep these groups alive and active.

▾ Remind yourself of what you are fighting for by going out to the wild places you love.

and try to leave the land in as good condition or better than when you found it is the land ethic incarnate.

But just as we can't separate Yellowstone Park from the land around it or the air that floats over the Colorado Plateau from the air in the cities of the Southwest, we can't separate our good deeds in the woods from our lives back home. The wild places that resuscitate minds and give life to our spirits exist only because our forebears, John Muir, Aldo Leopold, Rosalie Edge and the rest, had the foresight and the guts to defend them. The wilds that remain will stay wild only because we, the body politic, insist on it.

The land ethic isn't something to be put in the closet and stored like some sleeping bag when we finish the trip at the parking lot. At home, back in the cities, we need to be advocates for the wild areas and use our political powers to protect the wild areas we love. One needn't be righteous or shrill about one's land ethic. We're all dependent to one degree or another on the same economic system and the same extractive industries. It's nearly impossible not to be. As Thomas McGuane said in his essay "On the Henry's Fork," "... human lives are swept along by fear and need and creaturely habit."* I think the best, most effective conservationists I know have deep beliefs and an abiding passion about saving the wild places; but they are sustained by humor and irony.

*Thomas McGuane, *Heart of the Land,* edited by Joseph Barbato and Lisa Weinerman, Vintage Books, 1996, p. 54.

I'm certainly no angel when it comes to consuming my share of the world's resources and use plenty of petroleum-based products and wood that may have come from a forest better left untouched. The challenge, though, is to start with the presumption that certain parts of the earth should be protected and kept in their natural state no matter what. The challenge is to work backward from that assumption: to set limits on where we go with our roads and machines and developments and manage to make a collective living despite those limits.

On NOLS courses we try to teach students to be responsible to the land by camping with a light touch and camping thoughtfully. Our hopes are that those habits will be transferred to their lives when they return to the city—that they will do small and great things to preserve the natural places. Some of our students—Pamela Eaton, for example—have gone on to do work that has made a thunderclapping difference.

Here's hoping that you, a person who presumably loves the outdoors, will put your own energies and talents to preserving the places you love. And here's hoping that you get to enjoy those places with skills you have learned from this book.

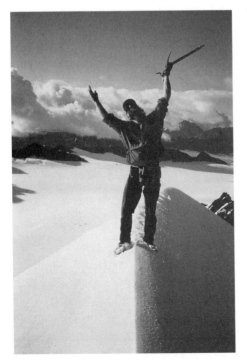

Whiteout Peak in Alaska's Chugach Range. *Deborah Sussex*

# Equipment List

**FOOTWEAR**

Socks, 3 to 5 pairs of wool or synthetic material
Hiking boots, 1 pair
Camp shoes, 1 pair
Gaiters, 1 pair, long

**UPPER BODY LAYERS**

You should have at least three insulating layers that can be worn comfortably together. If you do not stay warm easily or are traveling in the spring or fall, you may want to bring four insulating layers.

**Base layer:** This layer goes against your skin and should be made of a material that keeps you warm even when wet. The layer will wick water away from your skin and dry quickly as well. Choose one of the following:

Lightweight high-performance polyester shirt
Polypropylene shirt
Capilene shirt
Light wool shirt

**Intermediate layers:** The intermediate layers insulate. We recommend a midweight intermediate layer such as a pile shirt and a heavy intermediate layer such as a pile jacket. Choose at least one layer from the list of midweight articles and one layer from the list of heavyweight articles:

Midweight
    Midweight wool shirt
    Sweater
    Pile shirt (Polartec 100 weight)

Heavyweight
    Heavyweight pile jacket
    Heavy wool sweater
    Down or fiberfill jacket

**Outer layer:** The outer layers must protect you from the heat loss associated with convection and from rain or snow as well. Two layers—one breathable and the other waterproof—are best.

Wind shirt: A lightweight, breathable garment that will fit over three layers of insulation. Uncoated nylon or lightweight Gore-Tex is acceptable.

Waterproof cagoule or storm jacket: A durable, lightweight waterproof garment that will fit over three layers of insulation. This layer can be made of coated nylon or Gore-Tex.

1 cotton T-shirt

### LOWER BODY LAYERS

Nylon hiking shorts
Wind pants
Lightweight or midweight long underwear bottoms
Pile pants for staying warm at night (optional)

### BACKPACK AND STORAGE BAGS

Backpack (with a volume between 4,000 and 7,500 cubic inches)
Day pack (with a volume between 1,500 and 3,000 cubic inches)
2 nylon zip bags for packing food and clothing (approximately 12" x 24")
Large stuff sack or compression sack for sleeping bag
2 to 3 small stuff sacks to organize gear
2 large garbage bags (for waterproofing sleeping bag and clothing bag)

## SLEEPING GEAR

Sleeping bag

Sleeping pad (closed-cell foam or lightweight air mattress–style)

Ground cloth (for sleeping outside the tent or if using only a fly)

## HATS AND GLOVES

Baseball cap or golf hat for sun protection

Wool or pile hat

One pair of gloves (wool or synthetic). In the spring or fall, consider bringing two pairs.

Balaclava (optional for areas with harsher climate or during the spring and fall)

## MISCELLANEOUS PERSONAL GEAR

Eating utensils: 1 each: cup, bowl, and spoon. Insulated mug with lid (12 oz. or larger).

Water bottle or wide-mouth bottle with 1-quart capacity

Lip balm: stick, cream, or tube with sun protection factor (SPF) of 15 or more

Sunscreen: SPF factor of 15 or more

Bandannas: 1 or 2 for washing face, makeshift splints, sun protection, etc.

Sunglasses: should block 100 percent of ultraviolet light and 95 percent of infrared light. Side shields recommended for snow or glacier travel. Bring a sturdy case.

Headlamp or flashlight: Bring an extra set of batteries and an extra bulb.

Disposable lighter: Bring two to light stoves and fires. The waterproof ones are more expensive but are also more reliable.

Toilet articles: toothbrush, toothpaste, comb, tampons, medication (if applicable)

Underwear: two changes. Most women prefer jogbras.

Prescription glasses or contact lenses: If you wear glasses bring a backup pair, and if you wear contacts bring a pair of glasses as well.

Notebook and pens/pencils. A small, light pad is nice to have if you care to keep a journal or to sketch. Paper is always useful if you have to send out instructions for an evacuation.

Watch

Pocketknife or multipurpose tool: for cleaning fish, preparing food, and repairing gear.

## G R O U P   G E A R

Tent or fly
Camp stove and fuel bottles
First aid kit (see page 214)
Cooking gear
 4-quart pot
 fry pan (optional)
 large cooking spoon
 large metal or plastic ladle
 spatula (optional)
 pair of pot grips (a small pair of channel-lock pliers works well)
 large water vessel (2 to 4 gallon capacity) to haul water to camp kitchen
Small trowel to dig cathole for human waste
Maps and compass
Binoculars
Reference books or field guides
Water filter/purifier
Bear hanging gear or bear-resistant food containers
Fishing gear
Repair kit
 Speedy stitcher
 Toggles
 Ripstop nylon repair tape, 2 feet
 Parachute cord, 20 feet
 Tent pole splint, 1 each
 Duct tape, 1 small roll
 Sewing kit
 Barge cement, 1 can
 Wire, 10 feet

# Suggested Reading

Fleming, June. *Staying Found: The Complete Map and Compass Handbook,* 2nd ed. Seattle: The Mountaineers, 1994.

Fletcher, Colin. *The Complete Walker.* New York: Alfred A. Knopf, 1984.

Graydon, Don, ed. *Mountaineering: The Freedom of the Hills.* Seattle: The Mountaineers, 1992.

Hampton, Bruce, and David Cole. *Soft Paths,* 2nd ed. Harrisburg, Pa.: Stackpole Books, 1995.

Krutch, Joseph Wood. *The Best Nature Writing of Joseph Wood Krutch.* 1949. Reprint, with a foreword by Edward Lueders, Salt Lake City: University of Utah Press, 1995.

Leopold, Aldo. *A Sand County Almanac.* 1949. Reprint, with an introduction by Robert Finch, Oxford: Oxford University Press, 1989.

Pearson, Claudia, ed. *The NOLS Cookery,* 4th ed. Harrisburg, Pa.: Stackpole Books, 1997.

Petzoldt, Paul. *The New Wilderness Handbook,* 2nd ed. New York: Norton, 1984.

Powers, Phil. *NOLS Wilderness Mountaineering.* Mechanicsburg, Pa.: Stackpole Books, 1993.

Seidman, David. *The Essential Wilderness Navigator: How to Find Your Way in the Great Outdoors.* Camden, Maine: The McGraw-Hill Companies, Ragged Mountain Press, 1995.

Shimelpfenig, Tod, and Linda Lindsey. *NOLS Wilderness First Aid.* Harrisburg, Pa.: Stackpole Books, 1992.

Stegner, Wallace. *Marking the Sparrow's Fall: Wallace Stegner's American West*. Edited by Page Stegner. New York: Henry Holt, 1998.

Wilkerson, James A., ed. *Medicine for Mountaineering*, 4th ed. Seattle: The Mountaineers, 1992.

# Index